R4

Books should be returned to the SDH Library on or before
the date stamped above unless a renewal has been arranged

Salisbury District Hospital Library

Telephone: Salisbury (01722) 336262 extn. 4432 / 33
Out of hours answer machine in operation

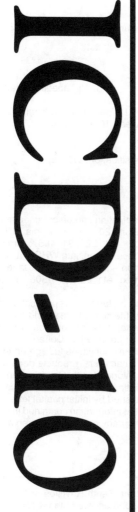

International Statistical Classification of Diseases and Related Health Problems

Tenth Revision

Volume 2
Instruction manual

Second Edition

World Health Organization
Geneva
2004

WHO Library Cataloguing-in-Publication Data

ICD-10 : international statistical classification of diseases and related health problems : tenth revision. — 2nd ed.

3 v.

Contents: v. 1. Tabular list — v. 2. Instruction manual — v. 3. Alphabetical index.

I.Disease - classification 2.Classification. 3.Manuals I.World Health Organization
II.Title: International statistical classification of diseases : 10th revision
III.Title: ICD-10. Second edition.

ISBN 92 4 154649 2 (vol. 1) (NLM classification: WB 15)
92 4 154653 0 (vol. 2)
92 4 154654 9 (vol. 3)

The 43rd World Health Assembly in 1990 approved the Tenth Revision of the International Classification of Diseases (WHA 43.24) and endorsed the recommendation of the International Conference for the Tenth Revision of the ICD held in Geneva from 26 September to 2 October 1989 concerning the establishment of an updating process within the 10-year revision cycle.

This recommendation was put into motion at the annual meeting of WHO Collaborating Centres for the Family of International Classifications in Tokyo, Japan in 1996 and later a formal mechanism to guide the updating process was established. According to this updating mechanism minor updates are made each year while major updates are made, if required, every three years.

For more information regarding the updating process and a cumulative list of the updates please see http://www.who.int/classifications/. Future updates will also be posted on this site.

This Second Edition of ICD-10 includes the corrigenda to Volume 1 which appeared as an addendum to Volume 3 of the first edition, as well as the updates that came into effect between 1998 and 2003.

Typeset by DIMDI in Germany
Printed in Switzerland

9 789241 546539

Contents

1. Introduction

This volume of the Tenth Revision of the International Statistical Classification of Diseases and Related Health Problems (ICD-10) contains guidelines for recording and coding, together with much new material on practical aspects of the classification's use, as well as an outline of the historical background to the classification. This material is presented as a separate volume for ease of handling when reference needs to be made at the same time to the classification (Volume 1) and the instructions for its use. Detailed instructions on the use of the Alphabetical Index are contained in the introduction to Volume 3.

This manual provides a basic description of the ICD, together with practical instructions for mortality and morbidity coders, and guidelines for the presentation and interpretation of data. It is not intended to provide detailed training in the use of the ICD. The material included here needs to be augmented by formal courses of instruction allowing extensive practice on sample records and discussion of problems.

If problems arising from the use of the ICD cannot be resolved either locally or with the help of national statistical offices, advice is available from the WHO Collaborating Centres for the Family of International Classifications (see Volume 1).

2. Description of the International Statistical Classification of Diseases and Related Health Problems

2.1 Purpose and applicability

A classification of diseases can be defined as a system of categories to which morbid entities are assigned according to established criteria. The purpose of the ICD is to permit the systematic recording analysis, interpretation and comparison of mortality and morbidity data collected in different countries or areas and at different times. The ICD is used to translate diagnoses of diseases and other health problems from words into an alphanumeric code, which permits easy storage, retrieval and analysis of the data.

In practice, the ICD has become the international standard diagnostic classification for all general epidemiological and many health management purposes. These include the analysis of the general health situation of population groups and the monitoring of the incidence and prevalence of diseases and other health problems in relation to other variables, such as the characteristics and circumstances of the individuals affected. The ICD is neither intended nor suitable for indexing of distinct clinical entities. There are also some constraints on the use of the ICD for studies of financial aspects, such as billing or resource allocation.

The ICD can be used to classify diseases and other health problems recorded on many types of health and vital records. Its original use was to classify causes of mortality as recorded at the registration of death. Later, its scope was extended to include diagnoses in morbidity. It is important to note that, although the ICD is primarily designed for the classification of diseases and injuries with a formal diagnosis, not every problem or reason for coming into contact with health services can be categorized in this way. Consequently, the ICD provides for a wide variety of signs, symptoms, abnormal findings, complaints, and social circumstances that may stand in place of a diagnosis on health-related records (see Volume 1, Chapters XVIII and XXI). It can therefore be used to classify data recorded under headings such as "diagnosis", "reason for admission", "conditions treated" and "reason for consultation", which appear on a wide variety of health records from which statistics and other health-situation information are derived.

2.2   The concept of a "family" of disease and health-related classifications

Although the ICD is suitable for many different applications, it does not serve all the needs of its various users. It does not provide sufficient detail for some specialties and sometimes information on different attributes of health conditions may be needed. ICD also is not useful to describe functioning and disability as aspects of health, and does not include a full array of health interventions or reasons for encounter.

Foundations laid by the International Conference on ICD-10 in 1989 have provided the basis for the development of a "family" of health classifications (see Volume 1, Report on the International Conference for the Tenth Revision, section 6). Over the recent years through the use of the ICD and development of related WHO health classifications the concept of a "family" was further developed. Currently the "family" designates a suite of integrated classification products that share similar features and can be used singularly or jointly to provide information on different aspects of health and the health care system. For example the ICD as a reference classification is mainly used to capture information on mortality and morbidity. Additional aspects of health domains, functioning and disability have now been jointly classified in the International Classification of Functioning, Disability and Health (ICF). In general, the WHO Family of International Classifications aims to provide a conceptual framework of information dimensions which are related to health and health management.   In this way they establish a common language to improve communication and permit comparisons of data across countries' health care disciplines, services and time. The World Health Organization and the WHO-FIC Network strive to build the family of classifications so that it is based on sound scientific and taxonomic principles; is culturally appropriate and internationally applicable; and focuses on the multi-dimensional aspects of health so that it meets the needs of its different users.

The WHO Family of International Classifications (WHO-FIC) attempts to serve as the framework of international standards to provide the building blocks of health information systems. Figure 1 represents the types of classifications in the WHO-FIC.

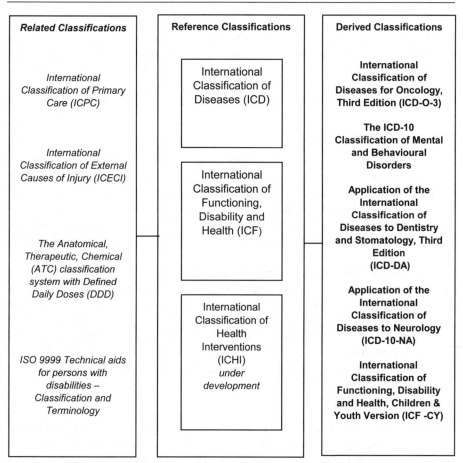

Figure 1: **Schematic representation of the WHO-FIC**

Reference classifications

These are the classifications that cover the main parameters of the health system, such as death, disease, functioning, disability, health and health interventions. WHO reference classifications are a product of international agreements. They have achieved broad acceptance and official agreement for use and are approved and recommended as guidelines for international reporting on health. They may be used as models for the development or revision of other classifications with respect to both the structure and the character and definition of the classes.

Currently there are two reference classifications in the WHO-FIC: ICD as a reference classification to capture information on mortality and morbidity and ICF to capture information on various domains of human functioning and disability. WHO has been exploring to the possibility of replacing the former International Classification of Procedures in Medicine (see below und non-diagnostic classifications) by a new International Classification of Health Interventions (ICHI). This process will take place over several stages of consultation, field testing and approval by the WHO governing bodies.

Derived classifications

Derived classifications are based upon reference classifications. Derived classifications may be prepared either by adopting the reference classification structure and classes, providing additional detail beyond that provided by the reference classification, or they may be prepared through rearrangement or aggregation of items from one or more reference classifications. Derived classifications are often tailored for use at the national or international level.

Within the WHO-FIC the derived classifications include specialty-based adaptations of ICF and ICD, such as the International Classification of Diseases for Oncology (ICD-O-3), the Application of the International Classification of Diseases to Dentistry and Stomatology, 3rd Edition (ICD-DA), the ICD-10 for Mental and Behavioural Disorders and the Application of the International Classification of Diseases to Neurology (ICD-10-NA) (see below under diagnosis-related classifications).

Related classifications

Related classifications are those that partially refer to reference classifications, or that are associated with the reference classification at specific levels of the structure only. Procedures for maintaining, updating and revising statistical classifications of the family encourage the resolution of problems of partial correspondence among related classifications, and offer opportunities for increased harmony over time. Within the WHO-FIC the related classifications include: the International Classification of Primary Care (ICPC-2), the International Classification of External Causes of Injury (ICECI), Technical aids for persons with disabilities: Classification and terminology (ISO9999) and the Anatomical Therapeutic Chemical Classification with Defined Daily Doses (ATC/DDD).

2.2.1 Diagnosis-related classifications

Special tabulation lists

The special tabulation lists are derived directly from the core classification, for use in data presentation and to facilitate analysis of health status and trends at the international, national and subnational levels. The special tabulation lists recommended for international comparisons and publications are included in Volume 1. There are five such lists, four for mortality and one for morbidity (for further details, see sections 5.4 and 5.5).

Specialty-based adaptations

Specialty-based adaptations usually bring together in a single, compact volume the sections or categories of the ICD that are relevant to a particular specialty. The four-character subcategories of the ICD are retained, but more detail is often given by means of fifth-character or sometimes sixth-character subdivisions, and there is an alphabetical index of relevant terms. Other adaptations may give glossary definitions of categories and subcategories within the specialty.

The adaptations have often been developed by international groups of specialists, but national groups have sometimes published adaptations that have later been used in other countries. The following list includes some of the major specialty adaptations to date.

Oncology

The third edition of the *International Classification of Diseases for Oncology* (ICD-O), published by WHO in 2000, is intended for use in cancer registries, and in pathology and other departments specializing in cancer (*1*). ICD-O is a dual-axis classification with coding systems for both topography and morphology. The topography code uses, for most neoplasms, the same three-character and four-character categories used in ICD-10 for malignant neoplasms (categories C00-C80). ICD-O thus allows greater specificity of site for non-malignant neoplasms than is possible in ICD-10.

The morphology code for neoplasms is identical to that in the *Systematized nomenclature of medicine* (SNOMED) (*2*), which was derived from the 1968 edition of the *Manual of tumor nomenclature and coding* (MOTNAC) (*3*) and the *Systematized nomenclature of pathology* (SNOP) (*4*). The morphology code has five digits; the first four digits identify the histological type and the fifth the behaviour of the neoplasm (malignant, *in situ*, benign, etc.). The ICD-O morphology code also appear in Volume 1 of ICD-10 and are added to the relevant entries in Volume 3, the Alphabetical Index. Tables are available for the conversion of the ICD-O third edition codes to ICD-10.

Dermatology

In 1978, the British Association of Dermatologists published the *International Coding Index for Dermatology* compatible with the Ninth Revision of the ICD. The Association has also published an adaptation of ICD-10 to dermatology, under the auspices of the International League of Dermatological Societies.

Dentistry and stomatology

The third edition of the Application of the International Classification of Diseases to Dentistry and Stomatology (ICD-DA), based on ICD-10, was published by WHO in 1995. It brings together ICD categories for diseases or conditions that occur in, have manifestations in, or have associations with the oral cavity and adjacent structures. It provides greater detail than ICD-10 by means of a fifth digit, but the numbering system is organized so that the relationship between an ICD-DA code and the ICD code from which it is derived is immediately obvious, and so that data from ICD-DA categories can be readily incorporated into ICD categories.

Neurology

In 1997 WHO published an adaptation of ICD-10 to neurology (ICD-NA), which retains the classification and coding systems of ICD-10 but is further subdivided at the fifth-character level and beyond to allow neurological diseases to be classified with greater precision.

Rheumatology and orthopaedics

The International League of Associations of Rheumatology is working on a revision of the Application of the International Classification of Diseases to Rheumatology and Orthopaedics (ICD-R&O), including the International Classification of Musculoskeletal Disorders (ICMSD), to be compatible with ICD-10. The ICD-R&O provides detailed specification of conditions through the use of additional digits, which allow for extra detail while retaining compatibility with ICD-10. The ICMSD is designed to clarify and standardize the use of terms and is supported by a glossary of generic descriptors for groups of conditions, such as the inflammatory polyarthropathies.

Paediatrics

Under the auspices of the International Pediatric Association, the British Paediatric Association (BPA) has published an application of ICD-10 to paediatrics, which uses a fifth digit to provide greater specificity. This follows similar applications prepared by BPA for ICD-8 and ICD-9.

Mental disorders

The ICD-10 Classification of Mental and Behavioural Disorders: clinical descriptions and diagnostic guidelines. This volume, published in 1992, provides for each category in Chapter V of ICD-10 (Mental and behavioural disorders) a general description and guidelines concerning the diagnosis, as well as comments about differential diagnosis and a listing of synonyms and exclusion terms (*5*). Where more detail is required, the guidelines give further subdivisions at the fifth and sixth digit levels. A second publication relating to Chapter V, *Diagnostic criteria for research*, was published in 1993.

A version of the classification for use in primary health care, and another version that uses a rearrangement of categories of childhood mental disorders in a multiaxial system, to allow simultaneous assessment of the clinical state, relevant environmental factors, and the degree of disability linked to the disease have also been developed.

2.2.2   Non-diagnostic classifications

Procedures in medicine

The *International Classification of Procedures in Medicine* (ICPM) was published in two volumes by WHO in 1978 (*6*). It includes procedures for medical diagnosis, prevention, therapy, radiology, drugs, and surgical and laboratory procedures. The classification has been adopted by some countries, while others have used it as a basis for developing their own national classifications of surgical operations.

The Heads of WHO Collaborating Centres for Classification of Diseases recognized that the process of consultation that had to be followed before finalization and publication was inappropriate in such a wide and rapidly advancing field. They therefore recommended that there should be no revision of the ICPM in conjunction with the Tenth Revision of the ICD.

In 1987, the Expert Committee on the International Classification of Diseases asked WHO to consider updating at least the outline for surgical procedures (Chapter 5) of the ICPM for the Tenth Revision. In response to this request and the needs expressed by a number of countries, the Secretariat prepared a tabulation list for procedures.

At their meeting in 1989, the Heads of the Collaborating Centres agreed that the list could serve as a guide for the national publication of statistics on surgical procedures and could also facilitate intercountry comparisons. The list could also be used as a basis for the development of comparable national classifications of surgical procedures.

Work on the list will continue, but any publication will follow the issue of ICD-10. In the meantime, other approaches to this subject are being explored. Some of these have common characteristics, such as a fixed field for specific items (organ, technique, approach, etc.), the possibility of being automatically updated, and the flexibility of being used for more than one purpose.

The International Classification of Functioning, Disability and Health

The International Classification of Functioning, Disability and Health (ICF) was published by WHO in all six WHO official languages in 2001, after its official endorsement by the Fifty-fourth World Health Assembly on 22 May 2001. It has subsequently been translated into over 25 languages.

ICF classifies health and health-related states in two parts. Part 1 classifies functioning and disability. Part 2 comprises environmental and personal contextual factors. Functioning and disability in Part 1 are described from the perspectives of the body, the individual, and society, formulated in two components: (1) body functions and structures, and (2) activities and participation. Since an individual's functioning and disability occur in a context, the ICF also includes a list of environmental factors.

The ICF has superseded the International Classification of Impairments, Disabilities and Handicaps (ICIDH). As a consequence the old ICIDH terms and definitions have been replaced by the following new ICF terms and definitions:

> *Functioning* is a generic term for body functions, body structures, activities and participation. It denotes the positive aspects of the interaction between an individual (with a health condition) and that individual's contextual factors (environmental and personal factors).

> *Disability* is an umbrella term for impairments, activity limitations and participation restrictions. It denotes the negative aspects of the interaction between an individual (with a health condition) and that individual's contextual factors (environmental and personal factors).

> *Body functions* are the physiological functions of body systems (including psychological functions).

Body structures are anatomical parts of the body such as organs, limbs and their components.

Impairments are problems in body function or structure such as a significant deviation or loss.

Activity is the execution of a task or action by an individual.

Activity limitations are difficulties an individual may have in executing activities.

Participation is involvement in a life situation.

Participation restrictions are problems an individual may experience in involvement in life situations.

Environmental factors make up the physical, social and attitudinal environment in which people live and conduct their lives.

ICF uses an alphanumeric system in which the letters *b*, *s*, *d* and *e* are used to denote Body Functions, Body Structures, Activities and Participation, and Environmental Factors. These letters are followed by a numeric code that starts with the chapter number (one digit), followed by the second level (two digits), and the third and fourth levels (one digit each). ICF categories are "nested" so that broader categories are defined to include more detailed subcategories of the parent category. Any individual may have a range of codes at each level. These may be independent or interrelated.

The ICF codes are only complete with the presence of a qualifier, which denotes a magnitude of the level of health (e.g. severity of the problem). Qualifiers are coded as one, two or more numbers after a point (or separator). Use of any code should be accompanied by at least one qualifier. Without qualifiers, codes have no inherent meaning. The first qualifier for Body Functions and Structures, the performance and capacity qualifiers for Activities and Participation, and the first qualifier for Environmental Factors all describe the extent of problems in the respective component.

The ICF puts the notions of 'health' and 'disability' in a new light. It acknowledges that every human being can experience a decrement in health and thereby experience some disability. This is not something that happens to only a minority of people. ICF thus 'mainstreams' the experience of disability and recognizes it as a universal human experience. By shifting the focus from cause to impact it places all health conditions on an equal footing allowing them to be compared using a common metric – the ruler of health and disability. Furthermore ICF takes into account the social aspects of disability and does not see disability only as a 'medical' or 'biological' dysfunction. By including Contextual Factors, in which environmental factors are listed, ICF allows the recording of the impact of the environment on the person's functioning.

The ICF is WHO's framework for measuring health and disability at both individual and population levels. While the International Classification of Diseases classifies diseases and causes of death, the ICF classifies health domains. The ICD and ICF constitute the two major building blocks of WHO's Family of International Classifications. Together, they provide exceptionally broad yet accurate tools to capture the full picture of health.

2.2.3 Information support to primary health care

One of the challenges of the Global Strategy for Health for All by the Year 2000 is to provide information support to primary health care (PHC). In countries without complete information or with only poor-quality data, a variety of approaches need to be adopted to supplement or replace the conventional use of the ICD.

Since the late 1970's, various countries have experimented with the collection of information by lay personnel. Lay reporting has subsequently been extended to a broader concept called "non-conventional methods". These methods, covering a variety of approaches, have evolved in different countries as a means of obtaining information on health status where conventional methods (censuses, surveys, vital or institutional morbidity and mortality statistics) have been found to be inadequate.

One of these approaches, "community-based information", involves community participation in the definition, collection and use of health-related data. The degree of community participation ranges from involvement only in data collection to the design, analysis and utilization of information. Experience in several countries has shown that this approach is more than a theoretical framework. The International Conference for the Tenth Revision of the International Classification of Diseases (see Volume 1) noted in its report:

> The Conference was informed about the experience of countries in developing and applying community-based health information that covered health problems and needs, related risk factors and resources. It supported the concept of developing non-conventional methods at the community level as a method of filling information gaps in individual countries and strengthening their information systems. It was stressed that, for both developed and developing countries, such methods or systems should be developed locally and that, because of factors such as morbidity patterns as well as language and cultural variations, transfer to other areas or countries should not be attempted.

Given the encouraging results of this approach in many countries, the Conference agreed that WHO should continue to give guidance on the development of local schemes and to support the progress of the methodology.

2.2.4   International Nomenclature of Diseases

In 1970, the Council for International Organizations of Medical Sciences (CIOMS) began the preparation of an International Nomenclature of Diseases (IND), with the assistance of its member organizations, and five volumes of provisional nomenclature were issued during 1972-1974. It was soon realized, however, that the compilation of such a nomenclature, were it to be truly international, would need much wider consultation than was possible through the members of CIOMS alone. In 1975, the IND became a joint project of CIOMS and WHO, guided by a Technical Steering Committee of representatives from both organizations.

The principal objective of the IND is to provide, for each morbid entity, a single recommended name. The main criteria for selection of this name are that it should be specific (applicable to one and only one disease), unambiguous, as self-descriptive as possible, as simple as possible, and (whenever feasible) based on cause. However, many widely used names that do not fully meet the above criteria are being retained as synonyms, provided they are not inappropriate, misleading, or contrary to the recommendations of international specialist organizations. Eponymous terms are avoided since they are not self-descriptive; however, many of these names are in such widespread use (e.g. Hodgkin disease, Parkinson disease and Addison disease) that they must be retained.

Each disease or syndrome for which a name is recommended is defined as unambiguously and as briefly as possible. A list of synonyms appears after each definition. These comprehensive lists are supplemented, if necessary, by explanations about why certain synonyms have been rejected or why an alleged synonym is not a true synonym.

The IND is intended to be complementary to the ICD. The differences between a nomenclature and a classification are discussed at 2.3. As far as possible, IND terminology has been given preference in the ICD.

The volumes of the IND published up to 1992 (*8*) are: *Infectious diseases* (bacterial diseases (1985), mycoses (1982), viral diseases (1983), parasitic diseases (1987)); *Diseases of the lower respiratory tract* (1979); *Diseases of the digestive system* (1990); *Cardiac and vascular diseases* (1989); *Metabolic, nutritional and endocrine disorders* (1991); *Diseases of the kidney, the lower urinary tract, and the male genital system* (1992); and *Diseases of the female genital system* (1992).

2.2.5   The role of WHO

Most of the classifications described above are the product of very close collaboration between nongovernmental organizations, other agencies, and divisions and units of WHO, with the unit responsible for the ICD and the ICF assuming a coordinating role and providing guidance and advice.

WHO promotes the development of adaptations that extend both the usefulness of the ICD and the ICF and the comparability of health statistics. The role of WHO in the development of new classifications, adaptations, and glossaries is to provide cooperative leadership and to act as a clearing-house, giving technical advice, guidance and support when needed. Anyone interested in preparing an adaptation of ICD-10 or the ICF should consult with WHO as soon as a clear statement of the objectives of the adaptation has been developed. Unnecessary duplication will thus be avoided by a coordinated approach to the development of the various components of the family.

2.3   General principles of disease classification

As William Farr stated in 1856 (*9*):

> Classification is a method of generalization. Several classifications may, therefore, be used with advantage; and the physician, the pathologist, or the jurist, each from his own point of view, may legitimately classify the diseases and the causes of death in the way that he thinks best adapted to facilitate his inquiries, and to yield general results.

A statistical classification of diseases must be confined to a limited number of mutually exclusive categories able to encompass the whole range of morbid conditions. The categories have to be chosen to facilitate the statistical study of disease phenomena. A specific disease entity that is of particular public health importance or that occurs frequently should have its own category. Otherwise, categories will be assigned to groups of separate but related conditions. Every disease or morbid condition must have a well defined place in the list of categories. Consequently, throughout the classification, there will be residual categories for other and miscellaneous conditions that cannot be allocated to the more specific categories. As few conditions as possible should be classified to residual categories.

It is the element of grouping that distinguishes a statistical classification from a nomenclature, which must have a separate title for each known morbid condition. The concepts of classification and nomenclature are nevertheless closely related because a nomenclature is often arranged systematically.

A statistical classification can allow for different levels of detail if it has a hierarchical structure with subdivisions. A statistical classification of diseases should retain the ability both to identify specific disease entities and to allow statistical presentation of data for broader groups, to enable useful and understandable information to be obtained.

The same general principles can be applied to the classification of other health problems and reasons for contact with health care services, which are also incorporated in the ICD.

The ICD has developed as a practical, rather than a purely theoretical classification, in which there are a number of compromises between classification based on etiology, anatomical site, circumstances of onset, etc. There have also been adjustments to meet the variety of statistical applications for which the ICD is designed, such as mortality, morbidity, social security and other types of health statistics and surveys.

2.4   The basic structure and principles of classification of the ICD

The ICD is a variable-axis classification. The structure has developed out of that proposed by William Farr in the early days of international discussions on classification structure. His scheme was that, for all practical, epidemiological purposes, statistical data on diseases should be grouped in the following way:

- epidemic diseases
- constitutional or general diseases
- local diseases arranged by site
- developmental diseases
- injuries.

This pattern can be identified in the chapters of ICD-10. It has stood the test of time and, though in some ways arbitrary, is still regarded as a more useful structure for general epidemiological purposes than any of the alternatives tested.

The first two, and the last two, of the groups listed above comprise "special groups", which bring together conditions that would be inconveniently arranged for epidemiological study were they to be scattered, for instance in a classification arranged primarily by anatomical site. The remaining group, "local diseases arranged by site", includes the ICD chapters for each of the main body systems.

The distinction between the "special groups" chapters and the "body systems" chapters has practical implications for understanding the structure of the classification, for coding to it, and for interpreting statistics based on it. It has to be remembered that, *in general*, conditions are primarily classified to one of the "special groups" chapters. Where there is any doubt as to where a condition should be positioned, the "special groups" chapters should take priority.

The basic ICD is a single coded list of three-character categories, each of which can be further divided into up to ten four-character subcategories. In place of the purely numeric coding system of previous revisions, the Tenth Revision uses an alphanumeric code with a letter in the first position and a number in the second, third and fourth positions. The fourth character follows a decimal point. Possible code numbers therefore range from A00.0 to Z99.9. The letter U is not used (see 2.4.7).

2.4.1   Volumes

ICD-10 comprises three volumes: Volume 1 contains the main classifications; Volume 2 provides guidance to users of the ICD; and Volume 3 is the Alphabetical Index to the classification.

Most of Volume 1 is taken up with the main classification, composed of the list of three-character categories and the tabular list of inclusions and four-character subcategories. The "core" classification - the list of three-character categories (Volume 1) - is the mandatory level for reporting to the WHO mortality database and for general international comparisons. This core classification also lists chapter and block titles. The tabular list, giving the full detail of the four-character level, is divided into 21 chapters.

Volume 1 also contains the following:

- *Morphology of neoplasms.* The classification of morphology of neoplasms may be used, if desired, as an additional code to classify the morphological type for neoplasms which, with a few exceptions, are classified in Chapter II only according to behaviour and site (topography). The morphology codes are the same as those used in the special adaptation of the ICD for oncology (ICD-O) (*1*).

- *Special tabulation lists*. Because the full four-character list of the ICD, and even the three-character list, are too long to be presented in every statistical table, most routine statistics use a tabulation list that emphasizes certain single conditions and groups others. The four special lists for the tabulation of mortality are an integral part of the ICD. Lists 1 and 2 are for general mortality and lists 3 and 4 are for infant and child mortality (ages 0 - 4 years). There is also a special tabulation list for morbidity. These are set out in Volume 1. Guidance on the appropriate use of the various levels of the classification and the tabulation lists is given in section 5 of this volume.
- *Definitions*. The definitions in Volume 1 have been adopted by the World Health Assembly and are included to facilitate the international comparability of data.
- *Nomenclature regulations*. The regulations adopted by the World Health Assembly set out the formal responsibilities of WHO Member States regarding the classification of diseases and causes of death, and the compilation and publication of statistics. They are found in Volume 1.

2.4.2   Chapters

The classification is divided into 21 chapters. The first character of the ICD code is a letter, and each letter is associated with a particular chapter, except for the letter D, which is used in both Chapter II, Neoplasms, and Chapter III, Diseases of the blood and blood-forming organs and certain disorders involving the immune mechanism, and the letter H, which is used in both Chapter VII, Diseases of the eye and adnexa and Chapter VIII, Diseases of the ear and mastoid process. Four chapters (Chapters I, II, XIX, and XX) use more than one letter in the first position of their codes.

Each chapter contains sufficient three-character categories to cover its content; not all available codes are used, allowing space for future revision and expansion.

Chapters I to XVII relate to diseases and other morbid conditions, and Chapter XIX to injuries, poisoning and certain other consequences of external causes. The remaining chapters complete the range of subject matter nowadays included in diagnostic data. Chapter XVIII covers Symptoms, signs and abnormal clinical and laboratory findings, not elsewhere classified. Chapter XX, External causes of morbidity and mortality, was traditionally used to classify causes of injury and poisoning, but, since the Ninth Revision, has also provided for any recorded external cause of diseases and other morbid conditions. Finally, Chapter XXI, Factors influencing health status and contact with health services, is intended for the classification of data explaining the reason for contact with health care services of a person not currently sick, or the circumstances in which the patient is receiving care at that particular time or otherwise having some bearing on that person's care.

2.4.3 Blocks of categories

The chapters are subdivided into homogeneous "blocks" of three-character categories. In Chapter I, the block titles reflect two axes of classification - mode of transmission and broad group of infecting organisms. In Chapter II, the first axis is the behaviour of the neoplasm; within behaviour, the axis is mainly by site, although a few three-character categories are provided for important morphological types (e.g. leukaemias, lymphomas, melanomas, mesotheliomas, Kaposi's sarcoma). The range of categories is given in parentheses after each block title.

2.4.4 Three-character categories

Within each block, some of the three-character categories are for single conditions, selected because of their frequency, severity or susceptibility to public health intervention, while others are for groups of diseases with some common characteristic. There is usually provision for "other" conditions to be classified, allowing many different but rarer conditions, as well as "unspecified" conditions, to be included.

2.4.5 Four-character subcategories

Although not mandatory for reporting at the international level, most of the three-character categories are subdivided by means of a fourth, numeric character after a decimal point, allowing up to ten subcategories. Where a three-character category is not subdivided, it is recommended that the letter "X" be used to fill the fourth position so that the codes are of a standard length for data-processing.

The four-character subcategories are used in whatever way is most appropriate, identifying, for example, different sites or varieties if the three-character category is for a single disease, or individual diseases if the three-character category is for a group of conditions.

The fourth character .8 is generally used for "other" conditions belonging to the three-character category, and .9 is mostly used to convey the same meaning as the three-character category title, without adding any additional information.

When the same fourth-character subdivisions apply to a range of three-character categories, they are listed once only, at the start of the range. A note at each of the relevant categories indicates where the details are to be found. For example, categories O03-O06, for different types of abortion, have common fourth characters relating to associated complications (see Volume 1).

2.4.6 Supplementary subdivisions for use at the fifth or subsequent character level

The fifth and subsequent character levels are usually subclassifications along a different axis from the fourth character. They are found in:

Chapter XIII - subdivisions by anatomical site

Chapter XIX - subdivisions to indicate open and closed fractures as well as intracranial, intrathoracic and intra-abdominal injuries with and without open wound

Chapter XX - subdivisions to indicate the type of activity being undertaken at the time of the event.

2.4.7 The unused "U" codes

Codes U00-U49 are to be used for the provisional assignment of new diseases of uncertain etiology. Codes U50-U99 may be used in research, e.g. when testing an alternative subclassification for a special project.

3. How to use the ICD

This section contains practical information which all users need to know in order to exploit the classification to its full advantage. Knowledge and understanding of the purpose and structure of the ICD are vital for statisticians and analysts of health information as well as for coders. Accurate and consistent use of the ICD depends on the correct application of all three volumes.

3.1 How to use Volume 1

3.1.1 Introduction

Volume 1 of the ICD contains the classification itself. It indicates the categories into which diagnoses are to be allocated, facilitating their sorting and counting for statistical purposes. It also provides those using statistics with a definition of the content of the categories, subcategories and tabulation list items they may find included in statistical tables.

Although it is theoretically possible for a coder to arrive at the correct code by the use of Volume 1 alone, this would be time-consuming and could lead to errors in assignment. An Alphabetical Index as a guide to the classification is contained in Volume 3. The Introduction to the Index provides important information about its relationship with Volume 1.

Most routine statistical uses of the ICD involve the selection of a single condition from a certificate or record where more than one is entered. The rules for this selection in relation to mortality and morbidity are contained in Section 4 of this Volume.

A detailed description of the tabular list is given in Section 2.4.

3.1.2   Use of the tabular list of inclusions and four-character subcategories

Inclusion terms

Within the three- and four-character rubrics[1], there are usually listed a number of other diagnostic terms. These are known as "inclusion terms" and are given, in addition to the title, as examples of the diagnostic statements to be classified to that rubric. They may refer to different conditions or be synonyms. They are not a subclassification of the rubric.

Inclusion terms are listed primarily as a guide to the content of the rubrics. Many of the items listed relate to important or common terms belonging to the rubric. Others are borderline conditions or sites listed to distinguish the boundary between one subcategory and another. The lists of inclusion terms are by no means exhaustive and alternative names of diagnostic entities are included in the Alphabetical Index, which should be referred to first when coding a given diagnostic statement.

It is sometimes necessary to read inclusion terms in conjunction with titles. This usually occurs when the inclusion terms are elaborating lists of sites or pharmaceutical products, where appropriate words from the title (e.g. "malignant neoplasm of ...", "injury to ...", "poisoning by ...") need to be understood.

General diagnostic descriptions common to a range of categories, or to all the subcategories in a three-character category, are to be found in notes headed "Includes", immediately following a chapter, block or category title.

Exclusion terms

Certain rubrics contain lists of conditions preceded by the word "Excludes". These are terms which, although the rubric title might suggest that they were to be classified there, are in fact classified elsewhere. An example of this is in category A46, "Erysipelas", where postpartum or puerperal erysipelas is excluded. Following each excluded term, in parentheses, is the category or subcategory code elsewhere in the classification to which the excluded term should be allocated.

---

[1] In the context of the ICD, "rubric" denotes either a three-character category or a four-character subcategory.

General exclusions for a range of categories or for all subcategories in a three-character category are to be found in notes headed "Excludes", immediately following a chapter, block or category title.

Glossary descriptions

In addition to inclusion and exclusion terms, Chapter V, Mental and behavioural disorders, uses glossary descriptions to indicate the content of rubrics. This device is used because the terminology of mental disorders varies greatly, particularly between different countries, and the same name may be used to describe quite different conditions. The glossary is not intended for use by coding staff.

Similar types of definition are given elsewhere in the ICD, for example, Chapter XXI, to clarify the intended content of a rubric.

3.1.3   Two codes for certain conditions

The "dagger and asterisk" system

ICD-9 introduced a system, continued in ICD-10, whereby there are two codes for diagnostic statements containing information about both an underlying generalized disease and a manifestation in a particular organ or site which is a clinical problem in its own right.

The primary code is for the underlying disease and is marked with a dagger (†); an optional additional code for the manifestation is marked with an asterisk (*). This convention was provided because coding to underlying disease alone was often unsatisfactory for compiling statistics relating to particular specialties, where there was a desire to see the condition classified to the relevant chapter for the manifestation when it was the reason for medical care.

While the dagger and asterisk system provides alternative classifications for the presentation of statistics, it is a principle of the ICD that the dagger code is the primary code and must always be used. Provision should be made for the asterisk code to be used *in addition* if the alternative method of presentation may also be required. For coding, the asterisk code must never be used alone. Statistics incorporating the dagger codes conform with the traditional classification for presenting data on mortality and morbidity and other aspects of medical care.

Asterisk codes appear as three-character categories. There are separate categories for the same conditions occurring when a particular disease is not specified as the underlying cause. For example, categories G20 and G21 are for forms of Parkinsonism that are not manifestations of other diseases assigned elsewhere, while category G22* is for "Parkinsonism in diseases classified elsewhere". Corresponding dagger codes are given for conditions mentioned in asterisk categories; for example, for Syphilitic parkinsonism in G22*, the dagger code is A52.1†.

Some dagger codes appear in special dagger categories. More often, however, the dagger code for dual-element diagnoses and unmarked codes for single-element conditions may be derived from the same category or subcategory.

The areas of the classification where the dagger and asterisk system operates are limited; there are 83 special asterisk categories throughout the classification, which are listed at the start of the relevant chapters.

Rubrics in which dagger-marked terms appear may take one of three different forms:

(i)   If the symbol (†) and the alternative asterisk code both appear in the rubric heading, all terms classifiable to that rubric are subject to dual classification and all have the same alternative code, e.g.

      A17.0† Tuberculous meningitis (G01*)
             Tuberculosis of meninges (cerebral) (spinal)
             Tuberculous leptomeningitis

(ii)   If the symbol appears in the rubric heading but the alternative asterisk code does not, all terms classifiable to that rubric are subject to dual classification but they have different alternative codes (which are listed for each term), e.g.

      A18.1† Tuberculosis of genitourinary system
             Tuberculosis of:
- bladder (N33.0*)
- cervix (N74.0*)
- kidney (N29.1*)
- male genital organs (N51.-*)
- ureter (N29.1*)

             Tuberculous female pelvic inflammatory disease (N74.1*)

(iii)   If neither the symbol nor the alternative code appear in the title, the rubric as a whole is not subject to dual classification but individual inclusion terms may be; if so, these terms will be marked with the symbol and their alternative codes given, e.g.

> A54.8   Other gonococcal infections
> Gonococcal:
>
> ...
>
> - peritonitis† (K67.1*)
> - pneumonia† (J17.0*)
> - septicaemia
> - skin lesions

Other optional dual coding

There are certain situations, other than in the dagger and asterisk system, that permit two ICD codes to be used to describe fully a person's condition. The note in the tabular list, "Use additional code, if desired ...", identifies many of these situations. The additional codes would be used only in special tabulations.

These are:

(i)   for local infections, classifiable to the "body systems" chapters, codes from Chapter I may be added to identify the infecting organism, where this information does not appear in the title of the rubric. A block of categories, B95-B97, is provided for this purpose in Chapter I.

(ii)   for neoplasms with functional activity. To the code from Chapter II may be added the appropriate code from Chapter IV to indicate the type of functional activity.

(iii)   for neoplasms, the morphology code from Volume 1, although not part of the main ICD, may be added to the Chapter II code to identify the morphological type of the tumour.

(iv)   for conditions classifiable to F00-F09 (Organic, including symptomatic, mental disorders) in Chapter V, where a code from another chapter may be added to indicate the cause, i.e. the underlying disease, injury or other insult to the brain.

(v)   where a condition is caused by a toxic agent, a code from Chapter XX may be added to identify that agent.

(vi)   where two codes can be used to describe an injury, poisoning or other adverse effect: a code from Chapter XIX, which describes the nature of the injury, and a code from Chapter XX, which describes the cause. The choice as to which code should be the additional code depends upon the purpose for which the data are being collected. (See introduction to Chapter XX, of Volume 1.)

3.1.4   Conventions used in the tabular list

In listing inclusion and exclusion terms in the tabular list, the ICD employs some special conventions relating to the use of parentheses, square brackets, colons, braces, the abbreviation "NOS", the phrase "not elsewhere classified" (NEC), and the word "and" in titles. These need to be clearly understood both by coders and by anyone wishing to interpret statistics based on the ICD.

Parentheses ( )

Parentheses are used in Volume 1 in four important situations.

(a)   Parentheses are used to enclose supplementary words, which may follow a diagnostic term without affecting the code number to which the words outside the parentheses would be assigned. For example, in I10 the inclusion term, "Hypertension (arterial) (benign) (essential) (malignant) (primary) (systemic)", implies that I10 is the code number for the word "Hypertension" alone or when qualified by any, or any combination, of the words in parentheses.

(b)   Parentheses are also used to enclose the code to which an exclusion term refers. For example,

H01.0 Blepharitis
        Excludes: blepharoconjunctivitis (H10.5).

(c)   Another use of parentheses is in the block titles, to enclose the three-character codes of categories included in that block.

(d)   The last use of parentheses was incorporated in the Ninth Revision and is related to the dagger and asterisk system. Parentheses are used to enclose the dagger code in an asterisk category or the asterisk code following a dagger term.

Square brackets [ ]

Square brackets are used:

(a)   for enclosing synonyms, alternative words or explanatory phrases; for example,

A30 Leprosy [Hansen's disease];

(b)   for referring to previous notes; for example,

C00.8 Overlapping lesion of lip [See note 5 at the beginning of this chapter];

(c)   for referring to a previously stated set of fourth character subdivisions common to a number of categories; for example,

K27 Peptic ulcer, site unspecified [See before K25 for subdivisions].

Colon :

A colon is used in listings of inclusion and exclusion terms when the words that precede it are not complete terms for assignment to that rubric. They require one or more of the modifying or qualifying words indented under them before they can be assigned to the rubric. For example, in K36, "Other appendicitis", the diagnosis "appendicitis" is to be classified there only if qualified by the words "chronic" or "recurrent".

Brace }

A brace is used in listings of inclusion and exclusion terms to indicate that neither the words that precede it nor the words after it are complete terms. Any of the terms before the brace should be qualified by one or more of the terms that follow it. For example:

O71.6   Obstetric damage to pelvic joints and ligaments
Avulsion of inner symphyseal cartilage
Damage to coccyx   obstetric
Traumatic separation of symphysis (pubis)

"NOS"

The letters NOS are an abbreviation for "not otherwise specified", implying "unspecified" or "unqualified".

Sometimes an unqualified term is nevertheless classified to a rubric for a more specific type of the condition. This is because, in medical terminology, the most common form of a condition is often known by the name of the condition itself and only the less common types are qualified. For example, "mitral stenosis" is commonly used to mean "rheumatic mitral stenosis". These inbuilt assumptions have to be taken into account in order to avoid incorrect classification. Careful inspection of inclusion terms will reveal where an assumption of cause has been made; coders should be careful not to code a term as unqualified unless it is quite clear that no information is available that would permit a more specific assignment elsewhere. Similarly, in interpreting statistics based on the ICD, some conditions assigned to an apparently specified category will not have been so specified on the record that was coded. When comparing trends over time and interpreting statistics, it is important to be aware that assumptions may change from one revision of the ICD to another. For example, before the Eighth Revision, an unqualified aortic aneurysm was assumed to be due to syphilis.

"Not elsewhere classified"

The words "not elsewhere classified", when used in a three-character category title, serve as a warning that certain specified variants of the listed conditions may appear in other parts of the classification. For example:

> J16   Pneumonia due to other infectious organisms, not elsewhere classified

This category includes J16.0 Chlamydial pneumonia and J16.8 Pneumonia due to other specified infectious organisms. Many other categories are provided in Chapter X (for example, J10-J15) and other chapters (for example, P23.- Congenital pneumonia) for pneumonias due to specified infectious organisms. J18 Pneumonia, organism unspecified, accommodates pneumonias for which the infectious agent is not stated.

"And" in titles

"And" stands for "and/or". For example, in the rubric A18.0, Tuberculosis of bones and joints, are to be classified cases of "tuberculosis of bones", "tuberculosis of joints" and "tuberculosis of bones and joints".

Point dash.-

In some cases, the fourth character of a subcategory code is replaced by a dash, e.g.

> G03   Meningitis due to other and unspecified causes,
>   Excludes: meningoencephalitis (G04.-)

This indicates to the coder that a fourth character exists and should be sought in the appropriate category. This convention is used in both the tabular list and the alphabetical index.

3.1.5 Categories with common characteristics

For quality control it is useful to introduce programmed checks into the computer system. The following groups of categories are provided as a basis for such checks on internal consistency, grouped according to the special characteristic that unites them.

Asterisk categories

The following asterisk categories are not to be used alone; they must always be used in addition to a dagger code:

D63*, D77*, E35*, E90*, F00*, F02*, G01*, G02*, G05*, G07*, G13*, G22*, G26*, G32*, G46*, G53*, G55*, G59*, G63*, G73*, G94*, G99*, H03*, H06*, H13*, H19*, H22*, H28*, H32*, H36*, H42*, H45*, H48*, H58*, H62*, H67*, H75*, H82*, H94*, I32*, I39*, I41*, I43*, I52*, I68*, I79*, I98*, J17*, J91*, J99*, K23*, K67*, K77*, K87*, K93*, L14*, L45*, L54*, L62*, L86*, L99*, M01*, M03*, M07*, M09*, M14*, M36*, M49*, M63*, M68*, M73*, M82*, M90*, N08*, N16*, N22*, N29*, N33*, N37*, N51*, N74*, N77*, P75*

Categories limited to one sex

The following categories apply only to males:

B26.0, C60-C63, D07.4-D07.6, D17.6, D29.-, D40.-, E29.-, E89.5, F52.4, I86.1, L29.1, N40-N51, Q53-Q55, R86, S31.2-S31.3, Z12.5.

The following categories apply only to females:

A34, B37.3, C51-C58, C79.6, D06.-, D07.0-D07.3, D25-D28, D39.-, E28.-, E89.4, F52.5, F53.-, I86.3, L29.2, L70.5, M80.0-M80.1, M81.0-M81.1, M83.0, N70-N98, N99.2-N99.3, O00-O99, P54.6, Q50-Q52, R87, S31.4, S37.4-S37.6, T19.2-T19.3, T83.3, Y76.-, Z01.4, Z12.4, Z30.1, Z30.3, Z30.5, Z31.1, Z31.2, Z32-Z36, Z39.-, Z43.7, Z87.5, Z97.5.

Guidance for handling inconsistencies between conditions and sex is given at 4.2.5.

Sequelae categories

The following categories are provided for sequelae of conditions that are no longer in an active phase:

B90-B94, E64.-, E68, G09, I69.-, O97, T90-T98, Y85-Y89.

Guidance for coding sequelae for both mortality and morbidity purposes can be found at 4.2.4 and 4.4.2.

Postprocedural disorders

The following categories are not to be used for underlying-cause mortality coding. Guidance for their use in morbidity coding is found at 4.4.2.

E89.-, G97.-, H59.-, H95.-, I97.-, J95.-, K91.-, M96.-, N99.-.

3.2 How to use Volume 3

The Introduction to Volume 3, the Alphabetical Index to ICD-10, gives instructions on how to use it. These instructions should be studied carefully before starting to code. A brief description of the structure and use of the Index is given below.

3.2.1 Arrangement of the Alphabetical Index

Volume 3 is divided into three sections as follows:

- Section I lists all the terms classifiable to Chapters I-XIX and Chapter XXI, except drugs and other chemicals.
- Section II is the index of external causes of morbidity and mortality and contains all the terms classifiable to Chapter XX, except drugs and other chemicals.
- Section III, the Table of Drugs and Chemicals, lists for each substance the codes for poisonings and adverse effects of drugs classifiable to Chapter XIX, and the Chapter XX codes that indicate whether the poisoning was accidental, deliberate (self-harm), undetermined, or an adverse effect of a correct substance properly administered.

3.2.2   Structure

The Index contains "lead terms", positioned to the far left of the column, with other words ("modifiers" or "qualifiers") at different levels of indentation under them. In Section I, these indented modifiers or qualifiers are usually varieties, sites or circumstances that affect coding; in Section II they indicate different types of accident or occurrence, vehicles involved, etc. Modifiers that do not affect coding appear in parentheses after the condition.

3.2.3   Code numbers

The code numbers that follow the terms refer to the categories and subcategories to which the terms should be classified. If the code has only three characters, it can be assumed that the category has not been subdivided. In most instances where the category has been subdivided, the code number in the Index will give the fourth character. A dash in the fourth position (e.g. O03.-) means that the category has been subdivided and that the fourth character can be found by referring to the tabular list. If the dagger and asterisk system applies to the term, both codes are given.

3.2.4   Conventions

Parentheses

Parentheses are used in the Index in the same way as in Volume 1, i.e. to enclose modifiers.

"NEC"

NEC (not elsewhere classified) indicates that specified variants of the listed condition are classified elsewhere, and that, where appropriate, a more precise term should be looked for in the Index.

Cross-references

Cross-references are used to avoid unnecessary duplication of terms in the Index. The word "see" requires the coder to refer to the other term; "see also" directs the coder to refer elsewhere in the Index if the statement being coded contains other information that is not found indented under the term to which "see also" is attached.

3.3   Basic coding guidelines

The Alphabetical Index contains many terms not included in Volume 1, and coding requires that both the Index and the Tabular List should be consulted before a code is assigned.

Before attempting to code, the coder needs to know the principles of classification and coding and to have carried out practical exercises.

The following is a simple guide intended to assist the occasional user of the ICD.

1. Identify the type of statement to be coded and refer to the appropriate section of the Alphabetical Index. (If the statement is a disease or injury or other condition classifiable to Chapters I - XIX or XXI, consult Section I of the Index. If the statement is the external cause of an injury or other event classifiable to Chapter XX, consult Section II.)

2. Locate the lead term. For diseases and injuries this is usually a noun for the pathological condition. However, some conditions expressed as adjectives or eponyms are included in the Index as lead terms.

3. Read and be guided by any note that appears under the lead term.

4. Read any terms enclosed in parentheses after the lead term (these modifiers do not affect the code number), as well as any terms indented under the lead term (these modifiers may affect the code number), until all the words in the diagnostic expression have been accounted for.

5. Follow carefully any cross-references ("see" and "see also") found in the Index.

6. Refer to the tabular list to verify the suitability of the code number selected. Note that a three-character code in the Index with a dash in the fourth position means that there is a fourth character to be found in Volume 1. Further subdivisions to be used in a supplementary character position are not indexed and, if used, must be located in Volume 1.

7. Be guided by any inclusion or exclusion terms under the selected code or under the chapter, block or category heading.

8. Assign the code.

Specific guidelines for the selection of the cause or condition to be coded, and for coding the condition selected, are given in Section 4.

4. Rules and guidelines for mortality and morbidity coding

This section concerns the rules and guidelines adopted by the World Health Assembly regarding the selection of a single cause or condition for routine tabulation from death certificates and morbidity records. Guidelines are also provided for the application of the rules and for coding of the condition selected for tabulation.

4.1 Mortality: guidelines for certification and rules for coding

Mortality statistics are one of the principal sources of health information and in many countries they are the most reliable type of health data.

4.1.1 Causes of death

In 1967, the Twentieth World Health Assembly defined the causes of death to be entered on the medical certificate of cause of death as "all those diseases, morbid conditions or injuries which either resulted in or contributed to death and the circumstances of the accident or violence which produced any such injuries". The purpose of the definition is to ensure that all the relevant information is recorded and that the certifier does not select some conditions for entry and reject others. The definition does not include symptoms and modes of dying, such as heart failure or respiratory failure.

When only one cause of death is recorded, this cause is selected for tabulation. When more than one cause of death is recorded, selection should be made in accordance with the rules given in section 4.1.5. The rules are based on the concept of the underlying cause of death.

4.1.2 Underlying cause of death

It was agreed by the Sixth Decennial International Revision Conference that the cause of death for primary tabulation should be designated the underlying cause of death.

From the standpoint of prevention of death, it is necessary to break the chain of events or to effect a cure at some point. The most effective public health objective is to prevent the precipitating cause from operating. For this purpose, the underlying cause has been defined as "(a) the disease or injury which initiated the train of morbid events leading directly to death, or (b) the circumstances of the accident or violence which produced the fatal injury".

4.1.3 International form of medical certificate of cause of death

The above principle can be applied uniformly by using the medical certification form recommended by the World Health Assembly. It is the responsibility of the medical practitioner signing the death certificate to indicate which morbid conditions led directly to death and to state any antecedent conditions giving rise to this cause.

The medical certificate shown below is designed to facilitate the selection of the underlying cause of death when two or more causes are recorded. Part I of the form is for diseases related to the train of events leading directly to death, and Part II is for unrelated but contributory conditions.

INTERNATIONAL FORM OF MEDICAL CERTIFICATE OF CAUSE OF DEATH

Cause of death		Approximate interval between onset and death
I Disease or condition directly leading to death*	(a) . . . . due to (or as a consequence of)	. . . .
Antecedent causes Morbid conditions, if any, giving rise to the above cause, stating the underlying condition last	(b) . . . . due to (or as a consequence of) (c) . . . . due to (or as a consequence of) (d)	. . . .
II Other significant conditions contributing to the death, but not related to the disease or condition causing it	. . . .	. . . .
*This does not mean the mode of dying, e.g. heart failure, respiratory failure. It means the disease, injury, or complication that caused death.		

The medical practitioner or other qualified certifier should use his or her clinical judgement in completing the medical certificate of cause of death. Automated systems must not include lists or other prompts to guide the certifier as these necessarily limit the range of diagnoses and therefore have an adverse effect on the accuracy and usefulness of the report.

In 1990, the Forty-third World Health Assembly adopted a recommendation that, where a need had been identified, countries should consider the possibility of an additional line, (d), in Part I of the certificate. However, countries may adopt, or continue to use, a certificate with only three lines in Part I where a fourth line is unnecessary, or where there are legal or other impediments to the adoption of the certificate shown above.

The condition recorded on the lowest used line of Part I of the certificate is usually the underlying cause of death used for tabulation. However, the procedures described in sections 4.1.4-4.1.5 may result in the selection of another condition as the underlying cause of death. To differentiate between these two possibilities, the expression *originating antecedent cause* (originating cause) will be used to refer to the condition proper to the last used line of Part I of the certificate, and the expression *underlying cause of death* will be used to identify the cause selected for tabulation.

If there is only one step in the chain of events, an entry at line I(a) is sufficient. If there is more than one step, the direct cause is entered at (a) and the originating antecedent cause is entered last, with any intervening cause entered on line (b) or on lines (b) and (c). An example of a death certificate with four steps in the chain of events leading directly to death is:

(a) Pulmonary embolism
(b) Pathological fracture
(c) Secondary carcinoma of femur
(d) Carcinoma of breast

Part II is for any other significant condition that contributed to the fatal outcome, but was not related to the disease or condition directly causing death.

After the words "due to (or as a consequence of)", which appear on the certificate, should be included not only the direct cause or pathological process, but also indirect causes, for example where an antecedent condition has predisposed to the direct cause by damage to tissues or impairment of function, even after a long interval.

Noting the approximate interval (minutes, hours, days, weeks, months or years) between the onset of each condition and the date of death helps the certifying doctor to establish the chain of events that led to the death, and is also useful subsequently in guiding the coder to choose the appropriate code.

In 1990, the World Health Assembly adopted a recommendation that countries should consider the inclusion on death certificates of questions about current pregnancy and pregnancy within one year preceding death.

4.1.4 Procedures for selection of the underlying cause of death for mortality tabulation

When only one cause of death is reported, this cause is used for tabulation.

When more than one cause of death is recorded, the first step in selecting the underlying cause is to determine the originating antecedent cause proper to the lowest used line in Part I of the certificate by application of the General Principle or of selection rules 1, 2 and 3.

In some circumstances the ICD allows the originating cause to be superseded by one more suitable for expressing the underlying cause in tabulation. For example, there are some categories for combinations of conditions, or there may be overriding epidemiological reasons for giving precedence to other conditions on the certificate.

The next step therefore is to determine whether one or more of the modification rules A to F (see section 4.1.9), which deal with the above situations, apply. The resultant code number for tabulation is that of the underlying cause.

Where the originating antecedent cause is an injury or other effect of an external cause classified to Chapter XIX, the circumstances that gave rise to that condition should be selected as the underlying cause for tabulation and coded to V01-Y89. The code for the injury or effect may be used as an additional code.

4.1.5 Rules for selection of the originating antecedent cause

Sequence

The term "sequence" refers to two or more conditions entered on successive lines of Part I, each condition being an acceptable cause of the one entered on the line above it.

Example 1:   I (a) Bleeding of oesophageal varices
                (b) Portal hypertension
                (c) Liver cirrhosis
                (d) Hepatitis B

If there is more than one cause of death in a line of the certificate, it is possible to have more than one reported sequence. In the example below, four sequences are reported:

Example 2:   I (a) Coma
                (b) Myocardial infarction and cerebrovascular accident
                (c) Atherosclerosis Hypertension

The sequences are:

- atherosclerosis (leading to) myocardial infarction (leading to) coma;
- atherosclerosis (leading to) cerebrovascular accident (leading to) coma;
- hypertension (leading to) myocardial infarction (leading to) coma;
- hypertension (leading to) cerebrovascular accident (leading to) coma;

General Principle

The General Principle states that when more than one condition is entered on the certificate, the condition entered alone on the lowest used line of Part I should be selected only if it could have given rise to all the conditions entered above it.

Selection rules

Rule 1. If the General Principle does not apply and there is a reported sequence terminating in the condition first entered on the certificate, select the originating cause of this sequence. If there is more than one sequence terminating in the condition mentioned first, select the originating cause of the first-mentioned sequence.

Rule 2. If there is no reported sequence terminating in the condition first entered on the certificate, select this first-mentioned condition.

Rule 3. If the condition selected by the General Principle or by Rule 1 or Rule 2 is obviously a direct consequence of another reported condition, whether in Part I or Part II, select this primary condition.

4.1.6   Some considerations on selection rules

In a properly completed certificate, the originating antecedent cause will have been entered alone on the lowest used line of Part I and the conditions, if any, that arose as a consequence of this initial cause will have been entered above it, one condition to a line in ascending causal order.

Example 3:   I (a) Uraemia
      (b) Hydronephrosis
      (c) Retention of urine
      (d) Hypertrophy of prostate

Example 4:   I (a) Bronchopneumonia
      (b) Chronic bronchitis
    II   Chronic myocarditis

In a properly completed certificate, therefore, the General Principle will apply. However, even if the certificate has not been properly completed, the General Principle may still apply provided that the condition entered alone on the lowest used line of Part I could have given rise to all the conditions above it, even though the conditions entered above it have not been entered in the correct causal order.

Example 5:   I (a) Generalized metastases   5 weeks
      (b) Bronchopneumonia   3 days
      (c) Lung cancer   11 months

The General Principle does not apply when more than one condition has been entered on the lowest used line of Part I, or if the single condition entered could not have given rise to all the conditions entered above it. Guidance on the acceptability of different sequences is given at the end of the rules, but it should be borne in mind that the medical certifier's statement reflects an informed opinion about the conditions leading to death and about their interrelationships, and should not be disregarded lightly.

Where the General Principle cannot be applied, clarification of the certificate should be sought from the certifier whenever possible, since the selection rules are somewhat arbitrary and may not always lead to a satisfactory selection of the underlying cause. Where further clarification cannot be obtained, however, the selection rules must be applied. Rule 1 is applicable only if there is a reported sequence, terminating in the condition first entered on the certificate. If such a sequence is not found, Rule 2 applies and the first-entered condition is selected.

The condition selected by the above rules may, however, be an obvious consequence of another condition that was not reported in a correct causal relationship with it, e.g. in Part II or on the same line in Part I. If so, Rule 3 applies and the originating primary condition is selected. It applies, however, only when there is no doubt about the causal relationship between the two conditions; it is not sufficient that a causal relationship between them would have been accepted if the certifier had reported it.

4.1.7   Examples of the General Principle and selection rules

General Principle

When more than one condition is entered on the certificate, select the condition entered alone on the lowest used line of Part I only if it could have given rise to all the conditions entered above it.

Example 6:   I (a)   Abscess of lung
              (b)   Lobar pneumonia

Select lobar pneumonia (J18.1).

Example 7:   I (a)   Hepatic failure
              (b)   Bile duct obstruction
              (c)   Carcinoma of head of pancreas

Select carcinoma of head of pancreas (C25.0).

Example 8:   I (a)   Cerebral haemorrhage
              (b)   Hypertension
              (c)   Chronic pyelonephritis
              (d)   Prostatic adenoma

Select prostatic adenoma (N40).

Example 9:   I (a)   Traumatic shock
              (b)   Multiple fractures
              (c)   Pedestrian hit by truck (traffic accident)

Select pedestrian hit by truck (V04.1).

Example 10:   I (a)   Bronchopneumonia
               II   Secondary anaemia and chronic lymphatic leukaemia

Select bronchopneumonia. But Rule 3 also applies; see Example 26.

Rule 1

If the General Principle does not apply and there is a reported sequence terminating in the condition first entered on the certificate, select the originating cause of this sequence. If there is more than one sequence terminating in the condition mentioned first, select the originating cause of the first-mentioned sequence.

Example 11: I (a) Bronchopneumonia
      (b) Cerebral infarction and hypertensive heart disease

Select cerebral infarction (I63.9). There are two reported sequences terminating in the condition first entered on the certificate; bronchopneumonia due to cerebral infarction, and bronchopneumonia due to hypertensive heart disease. The originating cause of the first-mentioned sequence is selected.

Example 12: I (a) Oesophageal varices and congestive heart failure
      (b) Chronic rheumatic heart disease and cirrhosis of liver

Select cirrhosis of liver (K74.6). The sequence terminating in the condition first entered on the certificate is oesophageal varices due to cirrhosis of liver.

Example 13: I (a) Acute myocardial infarction
      (b) Atherosclerotic heart disease
      (c) Influenza

Select atherosclerotic heart disease. The reported sequence terminating in the condition first entered on the certificate is acute myocardial infarction due to atherosclerotic heart disease. But Modification Rule C also applies; see Example 45.

Example 14: I (a) Pericarditis
      (b) Uraemia and pneumonia

Select uraemia. There are two reported sequences terminating in the condition first entered on the certificate: pericarditis due to uraemia and pericarditis due to pneumonia. The originating cause of the first-mentioned sequence is selected. But Modification Rule D also applies; see Example 60.

Example 15: I (a) Cerebral infarction and hypostatic pneumonia
      (b) Hypertension and diabetes
      (c) Atherosclerosis

Select atherosclerosis. There are two reported sequences terminating in the condition first entered on the certificate: cerebral infarction due to hypertension due to atherosclerosis and cerebral infarction due to diabetes. The originating cause of the first-mentioned sequence is selected. But Modification Rule C also applies; see Example 46.

Rule 2

If there is no reported sequence terminating in the condition first entered on the certificate, select this first-mentioned condition.

Example 16: I (a) Pernicious anaemia and gangrene of foot
 (b) Atherosclerosis

Select pernicious anaemia (D51.0). There is no reported sequence terminating in the first entered condition.

Example 17: I (a) Rheumatic and atherosclerotic heart disease

Select rheumatic heart disease (I09.9). There is no reported sequence; both conditions are on the same line.

Example 18: I (a) Fibrocystic disease of the pancreas
 (b) Bronchitis and bronchiectasis

Select fibrocystic disease of the pancreas (E84.9). There is no reported sequence.

Example 19: I (a) Senility and hypostatic pneumonia
 (b) Rheumatoid arthritis

Select senility. There is a reported sequence - hypostatic pneumonia due to rheumatoid arthritis - but it does not terminate in the condition first entered on the certificate. But Modification Rule A also applies; see Example 33.

Example 20: I (a) Bursitis and ulcerative colitis

Select bursitis. There is no reported sequence. But Modification Rule B also applies; see Example 41.

Example 21:   I (a)   Acute nephritis, scarlet fever.

Select acute nephritis. There is no reported sequence. But Rule 3 also applies; see Example 28.

Rule 3

If the condition selected by the General Principle or by Rule 1 or Rule 2 is obviously a direct consequence of another reported condition, whether in Part I or Part II, select this primary condition.

Assumed direct consequences of another condition

Kaposi's sarcoma, Burkitt's tumour and any other malignant neoplasm of lymphoid, haematopoietic and related tissue, classifiable to C46.- or C81-C96, should be considered to be a direct consequence of HIV disease, where this is reported. No such assumption should be made for other types of malignant neoplasm.

Any infectious disease classifiable to A00-B19, B25-B49, B58-B64, B99 or J12-J18 should be considered to be a direct consequence of reported HIV disease.

Certain postoperative complications (pneumonia (any type), haemorrhage, thrombophlebitis, embolism, thrombosis, septicaemia, cardiac arrest, renal failure (acute), aspiration, atelectasis and infarction) can be considered direct consequences of an operation, unless surgery was carried out four weeks or more before death.

Any pneumonia in J12-J18 should be considered an obvious consequence of conditions that impair the immune system. Pneumonia in J18.0 and J18.2-J18.9 should be considered an obvious consequence of wasting diseases (such as malignant neoplasm and malnutrition) and diseases causing paralysis (such as cerebral haemorrhage or thrombosis), as well as serious respiratory conditions, communicable diseases, and serious injuries. Pneumonia in J18.0 and J18.2-J18.9, J69.0, and J69.8 should also be considered an obvious consequence of conditions that affect the process of swallowing.

Any disease described or qualified as "embolic" may be assumed to be a direct consequence of venous thrombosis, phlebitis or thrombophlebitis, valvular heart disease, atrial fibrillation, childbirth or any operation.

Any disease described as secondary should be assumed to be a direct consequence of the most probable primary cause entered on the certificate.

Secondary or unspecified anaemia, malnutrition, marasmus or cachexia may be assumed to be a consequence of any malignant neoplasm.

Any pyelonephritis may be assumed to be a consequence of urinary obstruction from conditions such as hyperplasia of prostate or ureteral stenosis.

Nephritic syndrome may be assumed to be a consequence of any streptococcal infection (scarlet fever, streptococcal sore throat, etc.).

Dehydration may be assumed to be a consequence of any intestinal infectious disease.

An operation on a given organ should be considered a direct consequence of any surgical condition (such as malignant tumour or injury) of the same organ reported anywhere on the certificate.

Example 22: I (a) Kaposi's sarcoma
      II AIDS

      Select HIV disease resulting in Kaposi's sarcoma (B21.0)

Example 23: I (a) Cancer of ovary
      II HIV disease

      Select malignant neoplasm of ovary (C56)

Example 24: I (a) Tuberculosis
      II HIV disease

      Select HIV disease resulting in mycobacterial infection (B20.0)

Example 25: I (a) Cerebral toxoplasmosis and herpes zoster
       (b) Burkitt's lymphoma, HIV disease

      Select HIV disease resulting in multiple diseases classified elsewhere (B22.7). Cerebral toxoplasmosis, selected by Rule 2, can be considered a direct consequence of HIV disease.

Example 26: I (a) Bronchopneumonia
      II Secondary anaemia and chronic lymphatic leukaemia

      Select chronic lymphatic leukaemia (C91.1). Bronchopneumonia, selected by the General Principle (see Example 10), and secondary anaemia can both be considered direct sequels of chronic lymphatic leukaemia.

Example 27:   I (a) Cerebral haemorrhage
                 (b) Hypertension
                 (c) Chronic pyelonephritis and prostatic obstruction

Select prostatic obstruction (N40). Chronic pyelonephritis, selected by Rule 1, can be considered a direct sequel of prostatic obstruction.

Example 28:   I (a) Acute nephritis, scarlet fever

Select scarlet fever (A38). Acute nephritis, selected by Rule 2 (see Example 21), can be considered a direct sequel of scarlet fever.

Example 29:   I (a) Nephrectomy
                 II   Clear cell carcinoma of kidney

Select clear cell carcinoma of kidney (C64). There is no doubt that the nephrectomy was performed for the malignant neoplasm of kidney.

Example 30:   I (a) Acute anaemia
                 (b) Haematemesis
                 (c) Bleeding of oesophageal varices
                 (d) Portal hypertension
                 II   Cirrhosis of liver

Select cirrhosis of liver (K74.6). Portal hypertension, selected by the General Principle, can be considered a direct consequence of cirrhosis of liver.

Example 31:   I (a) Hypostatic pneumonia, cerebral
                 (b) Haemorrhage and cancer of breast

Select cerebral haemorrhage (I61.9). Hypostatic pneumonia, selected by Rule 2, can be considered a direct sequel of either of the other conditions reported; the one mentioned first is selected.

Example 32:   I (a) Pulmonary infarction
                 II   Left pneumonectomy for carcinoma of lung 3 weeks ago

Select carcinoma of lung (C34.9).

4.1.8   Modification of the selected cause

The selected cause of death is not necessarily the most useful and informative condition for tabulation. For example, if senility or some generalized disease such as hypertension or atherosclerosis has been selected, this is less useful than if a manifestation or result of aging or disease had been chosen. It may sometimes be necessary to modify the selection to conform with the requirements of the classification, either for a single code for two or more causes jointly reported or for preference for a particular cause when reported with certain other conditions.

The modification rules that follow are intended to improve the usefulness and precision of mortality data and should be applied after selection of the originating antecedent cause. The interrelated processes of selection and modification have been separated for clarity.

Some of the modification rules require further application of the selection rules, which will not be difficult for experienced coders, but it is important to go through the process of selection, modification and, if necessary, reselection.

4.1.9   The modification rules

Rule A. Senility and other ill-defined conditions

Where the selected cause is ill-defined and a condition classified elsewhere is reported on the certificate, reselect the cause of death as if the ill-defined condition had not been reported, except to take account of that condition if it modifies the coding. The following conditions are regarded as ill-defined: I46.9 (Cardiac arrest, unspecified); I95.9 (Hypotension, unspecified); I99 (Other and unspecified disorders of circulatory system); J96.0 (Acute respiratory failure); J96.9 (Respiratory failure, unspecified); P28.5 (Respiratory failure of newborn); R00-R94 and R96-R99 (Symptoms, signs and abnormal clinical and laboratory findings, not elsewhere classified). Note that R95 (Sudden infant death syndrome) is not regarded as ill-defined.

Rule B. Trivial conditions

Where the selected cause is a trivial condition unlikely to cause death and a more serious condition is reported, reselect the underlying cause as if the trivial condition had not been reported. If the death was the result of an adverse reaction to treatment of the trivial condition, select the adverse reaction.

Rule C. Linkage

Where the selected cause is linked by a provision in the classification or in the notes for use in underlying cause mortality coding with one or more of the other conditions on the certificate, code the combination.

Where the linkage provision is only for the combination of one condition specified as due to another, code the combination only when the correct causal relationship is stated or can be inferred from application of the selection rules.

Where a conflict in linkages occurs, link with the condition that would have been selected if the cause initially selected had not been reported. Make any further linkage that is applicable.

Rule D. Specificity

Where the selected cause describes a condition in general terms and a term that provides more precise information about the site or nature of this condition is reported on the certificate, prefer the more informative term. This rule will often apply when the general term becomes an adjective, qualifying the more precise term.

Rule E. Early and late stages of disease

Where the selected cause is an early stage of a disease and a more advanced stage of the same disease is reported on the certificate, code to the more advanced stage. This rule does not apply to a "chronic" form reported as due to an "acute" form unless the classification gives special instructions to that effect.

Rule F. Sequelae

Where the selected cause is an early form of a condition for which the classification provides a separate "Sequelae of ..." category, and there is evidence that death occurred from residual effects of this condition rather than from those of its active phase, code to the appropriate "Sequelae of ..." category.

"Sequelae of ..." categories are as follows: B90-B94, E64.-, E68, G09, I69, O97 and Y85-Y89.

4.1.10 Examples of the modification rules

Rule A. Senility and other ill-defined conditions

Where the selected cause is ill-defined and a condition classified elsewhere is reported on the certificate, reselect the cause of death as if the ill-defined condition had not been reported, except to take account of that condition if it modifies the coding. The following conditions are regarded as ill-defined: I46.9 (Cardiac arrest, unspecified); I95.9 (Hypotension, unspecified); I99 (Other and unspecified disorders of circulatory system); J96.0 (Acute respiratory failure); J96.9 (Respiratory failure, unspecified); P28.5 (Respiratory failure of newborn); R00–R94 and R96–R99 (Symptoms, signs and abnormal clinical and laboratory findings, not elsewhere classified). Note that R95 (Sudden infant death syndrome) is not regarded as ill-defined.

Example 33: I (a) Senility and hypostatic pneumonia
　　　　　　　　 (b) Rheumatoid arthritis

Code to rheumatoid arthritis (M06.9). Senility, selected by Rule 2 (see Example 19), is ignored and the General Principle applied.

Example 34: I (a) Anaemia
　　　　　　　　 (b) Splenomegaly

Code to splenomegalic anaemia (D64.8). Splenomegaly, selected by the General Principle, is ignored but modifies the coding.

Example 35: I (a) Myocardial degeneration and
　　　　　　　　 (b) emphysema
　　　　　　　　 (c) Senility

Code to myocardial degeneration (I51.5). Senility, selected by the General Principle, is ignored and Rule 2 applied.

Example 36: I (a) Cough and haematemesis

Code to haematemesis (K92.0). Cough, selected by Rule 2, is ignored.

Example 37: I (a) Terminal pneumonia
　　　　　　　　 (b) Spreading gangrene and cerebrovascular
　　　　　　　　 (c) infarction

Code to cerebrovascular infarction (I63.9). Gangrene, selected by Rule 1, is ignored and the General Principle is applied.

Rule B. Trivial conditions

Where the selected cause is a trivial condition unlikely to cause death and a more serious condition is reported, reselect the underlying cause as if the trivial condition had not been reported. If the death was the result of an adverse reaction to treatment of the trivial condition, select the adverse reaction.

Example 38:   I (a)   Dental caries
            II   Cardiac arrest

Code to cardiac arrest (I46.9). Dental caries, selected by the General Principle, is ignored.

Example 39:   I (a)   Ingrowing toenail and acute renal failure

Code to acute renal failure (N17.9). Ingrowing toenail, selected by Rule 2, is ignored.

Example 40:   I (a)   Intraoperative haemorrhage
              (b)   Tonsillectomy
              (c)   Hypertrophy of tonsils

Code to haemorrhage during surgical operation (Y60.0).

Example 41:   I (a)   Bursitis and ulcerative colitis

Code to ulcerative colitis (K51.9). Bursitis, selected by Rule 2 (see Example 20), is ignored.

Example 42:   I (a)   Paronychia
            II   Tetanus

Code to tetanus (A35). Paronychia, selected by the General Principle, is ignored.

Rule C. Linkage

Where the selected cause is linked by a provision in the classification or in the notes for use in underlying cause mortality coding with one or more of the other conditions on the certificate, code the combination.

Where the linkage provision is only for the combination of one condition specified as due to another, code the combination only when the correct

causal relationship is stated or can be inferred from application of the selection rules.

Where a conflict in linkages occurs, link with the condition that would have been selected if the cause initially selected had not been reported. Make any further linkage that is applicable.

Example 43:   I (a)   Intestinal obstruction
          (b)   Femoral hernia

Code to femoral hernia with obstruction (K41.3).

Example 44:   I (a)   Right bundle-branch block and Chagas' disease

Code to Chagas' disease with heart involvement (B57.2). Right bundle-branch block, selected by Rule 2, links with Chagas' disease.

Example 45:   I (a)   Acute myocardial infarction
          (b)   Atherosclerotic heart disease
          (c)   Influenza

Code to acute myocardial infarction (I21.9). Atherosclerotic heart disease, selected by Rule 1 (see Example 13), links with acute myocardial infarction.

Example 46:   I (a)   Cerebral infarction and hypostatic pneumonia
          (b)   Hypertension and diabetes
          (c)   Atherosclerosis

Code to cerebral infarction (I63.9). Atherosclerosis, selected by Rule 1 (see Example 15), links with hypertension, which itself links with cerebral infarction.

Example 47:   I (a)   Cardiac dilatation and renal sclerosis
          (b)   Hypertension

Code to hypertensive heart and renal disease (I13.9). All three conditions combine.

Example 48:   I (a)   Stroke
          (b)   Atherosclerosis and hypertensive heart
          (c)   disease

Code to hypertensive heart disease (I11.9). Atherosclerosis, selected by Rule 1, links with hypertensive heart disease since hypertensive heart disease would have been selected by the

General Principle if atherosclerosis had not been reported.

Example 49:   I (a)   Stroke and hypertensive
  (b)   heart disease
  (c)   Atherosclerosis

Code to stroke (I64). Atherosclerosis, selected by the General Principle, links with stroke since this condition would have been selected by Rule 2 if atherosclerosis had not been reported.

Example 50:   I (a)   Secondary polycythaemia
  (b)   Pulmonary emphysema
  (c)   Chronic bronchitis

Code to obstructive chronic bronchitis (J44.8).Chronic bronchitis, selected by the General Principle, links with emphysema.

Example 51:   I (a)   Cardiac dilatation
  (b)   Hypertension
  II   Atrophy of the kidneys

Code to hypertensive heart and renal disease I13.9. All three conditions combine.

Example 52:   I(a)   Bronchopneumonia (aspiration)
  (b)   Convulsions
  (c)   Tuberculous meningitis
  II   Pulmonary tuberculosis

Code to pulmonary tuberculosis (A16.2). Tuberculous meningitis, selected by the General Principle, is not to be used with mention of pulmonary tuberculosis.

Example 53:   I (a)   Occipital fracture
  (b)   Fall following epileptic convulsions

Code to epileptic convulsions (G40.9). Fall, selected by Rule 1, links with epileptic convulsions.

Example 54:   I (a)   Cardiac arrest
  II   Chagas' disease

Code to Chagas' disease with heart involvement (B57.2). Cardiac arrest, selected by the General Principle, links with Chagas' disease.

Rule D. Specificity

Where the selected cause describes a condition in general terms and a term that provides more precise information about the site or nature of this condition is reported on the certificate, prefer the more informative term. This rule will often apply when the general term becomes an adjective, qualifying the more precise term.

Example 55:   I (a) Cerebral infarction
                (b) Cerebrovascular accident

                  Code to cerebral infarction (I63.9).

Example 56:   I (a) Rheumatic heart disease, mitral stenosis

                  Code to rheumatic mitral stenosis (I05.0).

Example 57:   I (a) Meningitis
                (b) Tuberculosis

                  Code to tuberculous meningitis (A17.0). The conditions are stated in the correct causal relationship.

Example 58:   I (a) Severe hypertension in pregnancy
                II   Eclamptic convulsions

                  Code to eclampsia in pregnancy (O15.0).

Example 59:   I (a) Aneurysm of aorta
                (b) Syphilis

                  Code to syphilitic aneurysm of aorta (A52.0). The conditions are stated in the correct causal relationship.

Example 60:   I (a) Pericarditis
                (b) Uraemia and pneumonia

                  Code to uraemic pericarditis (N18.8). Uraemia, selected by Rule 1 (see Example 14), modifies the pericarditis.

Rule E. Early and late stages of disease

Where the selected cause is an early stage of a disease and a more advanced stage of the same disease is reported on the certificate, code to the more advanced stage. This rule does not apply to a "chronic" form reported as due to an "acute" form unless the classification gives special instructions to that effect.

Example 61:   I (a)   Tertiary syphilis
             (b)   Primary syphilis

Code to tertiary syphilis (A52.9).

Example 62:   I (a)   Eclampsia during pregnancy
             (b)   Pre-eclampsia

Code to eclampsia during pregnancy (O15.0).

Example 63:   I (a)   Chronic myocarditis
             (b)   Acute myocarditis

Code to acute myocarditis (I40.9).

Example 64:   I (a)   Chronic nephritis
             (b)   Acute nephritis

Code to chronic nephritis, unspecified (N03.9), as special instruction is given to this effect.

Rule F. Sequelae

Where the selected cause is an early form of a condition for which the classification provides a separate "Sequelae of ..." category, and there is evidence that death occurred from residual effects of this condition rather than from those of its active phase, code to the appropriate "Sequelae of ..." category.

"Sequelae of ..." categories are as follows: B90-B94, E64.-, E68, G09, I69, O97 and Y85-Y89.

Example 65:   I (a)   Pulmonary fibrosis
             (b)   Old pulmonary tuberculosis

Code to sequelae of respiratory tuberculosis (B90.9).

Example 66:   I(a)   Bronchopneumonia
             (b)   Curvature of spine
             (c)   Rickets in childhood

Code to sequelae of rickets (E64.3).

Example 67:   I (a)   Hydrocephalus
             (b)   Tuberculous meningitis

Code to sequelae of tuberculous meningitis (B90.0).

Example 68: I (a) Hypostatic pneumonia
        (b) Hemiplegia
        (c) Cerebrovascular accident (10 years)

Code to sequelae of cerebrovascular accident (I69.4).

Example 69: I (a) Chronic nephritis
        (b) Scarlet fever

Code to sequelae of other specified infectious and parasitic diseases (B94.8). The description of the nephritis as chronic implies that the scarlet fever is no longer in its active phase.

4.1.11 Notes for use in underlying cause mortality coding

The following notes often indicate that if the provisionally selected code, as indicated in the left-hand column, is present with one of the conditions listed below it, the code to be used is the one shown in bold type. There are two types of combination:

"with mention of" means that the other condition may appear anywhere on the certificate;

"when reported as the originating antecedent cause of" means that the other condition must appear in a correct causal relationship or be otherwise indicated as being "due to" the originating antecedent cause.

A00-B99   Certain infectious and parasitic diseases

Except for human immunodeficiency virus [HIV] disease (B20-B24), *when reported as the originating antecedent cause of* a malignant neoplasm, code **C00-C97**.

A15.-   Respiratory tuberculosis, bacteriologically and histologically confirmed

A16.-   Respiratory tuberculosis, not confirmed bacteriologically or histologically

with mention of:

J60-J64   (Pneumoconiosis), code **J65**

A17.-   Tuberculosis of nervous system

A18.-   Tuberculosis of other organs

with mention of:

A15 or A16 (Respiratory tuberculosis), code **A15, A16**, unless reported as the originating antecedent cause of and with a specified duration exceeding that of the condition in A15.- or A16.-

A39.2	Acute meningococcaemia
A39.3	Chronic meningococcaemia
A39.4	Meningococcaemia, unspecified

with mention of:

A39.0	(Meningococcal meningitis), code **A39.0**
A39.1	(Waterhouse-Friderichsen syndrome), code **A39.1**

A40.-	Streptococcal septicaemia
A41.-	Other septicaemia
A46	Erysipelas

Code to these diseases when they follow a superficial injury (any condition in S00, S10, S20, S30, S40, S50, S60, S70, S80, S90, T00, T09.0, T11.0), or first-degree burn; when they follow a more serious injury, code to the external cause of the injury.

B20-B24   Human immunodeficiency virus [HIV] disease

The subcategories at B20-B23 are the only optional four-character codes for countries using the four-character version of ICD-10. These four-character subcategories are provided for use where it is not possible or not desired to use multiple-cause coding.

Conditions classifiable to two or more subcategories of the same category should be coded to the .7 subcategory of the relevant category (B20 or B21). If desired, additional codes from within the block B20-B24 may be used to specify the individual conditions listed.

B22.7   HIV disease resulting in multiple diseases classified elsewhere

This subcategory should be used when conditions classifiable to two or more categories from B20-B22 are listed on the certificate. If desired, additional codes from within the block B20-B24 may be used to specify the individual conditions listed.

B95-B97   Bacterial, viral and other infectious agents

Not to be used for underlying cause mortality coding.

D50-D89	Diseases of the blood and blood-forming organs and certain disorders involving the immune mechanism

as the cause of:

B20-B24	Human immunodeficiency virus [HIV] disease and where the certificate indicates that the HIV disease is a result of a blood transfusion given as treatment for the originating condition, code **B20-B24**

E86	Volume depletion

with mention of:

A00-A09   (Intestinal infectious diseases), code **A00-A09**

E89.-	Postprocedural endocrine and metabolic disorders, not elsewhere classified

Not to be used for underlying cause mortality coding. See Operations, 4.2.6.

F01-F09	Organic, including symptomatic, mental disorders

Not to be used if the underlying physical condition is known.

F10-F19	Mental and behavioural disorders due to psychoactive substance use

Fourth characters .0 (Acute intoxication) and .5 (Psychotic disorder) *with mention of* Dependence syndrome (.2), code **F10-F19** with fourth character **.2**

F10.-	Mental and behavioural disorders due to use of alcohol

with mention of:

K70.- (Alcoholic liver disease), code **K70.-**

F10.2	Dependence syndrome due to use of alcohol

with mention of:

F10.4, F10.6, F10.7 Withdrawal state with delirium, Amnesic syndrome, Residual and late-onset psychotic disorder, code **F10.4, F10.6, F10.7**

F17.-   Mental and behavioural disorders due to use of tobacco

when reported as the originating antecedent cause of:

C34.-   (Malignant neoplasm of bronchus and lung), code **C34.-**

I20-I25   (Ischaemic heart disease), code **I20-I25**

J40-J47   (Chronic lower respiratory disease), code **J40-J47**

F70-F79   Mental retardation

Not to be used if the underlying physical condition is known

G25.5   Other chorea

with mention of:

I00-I02   (Acute rheumatic fever), code **I02.-**

I05-I09   (Chronic rheumatic heart disease), code **I02.-**

G81.-   Hemiplegia
G82.-   Paraplegia and tetraplegia
G83.-   Other paralytic syndromes

Not to be used if the cause of the paralysis is known.

G97.-   Postprocedural disorders of nervous system, not elsewhere classified

Not to be used for underlying cause mortality coding. See Operations, 4.2.6.

H54.-   Blindness and low vision

Not to be used if the antecedent condition is known.

H59.-   Postprocedural disorders of eye and adnexa, not elsewhere classified

Not to be used for underlying cause mortality coding. See Operations, 4.2.6.

H90.-   Conductive and sensorineural hearing loss
H91.-   Other hearing loss

Not to be used if the antecedent condition is known.

H95.-	Postprocedural disorders of ear and mastoid process, not elsewhere classified

Not to be used for underlying cause mortality coding. See Operations, 4.2.6.

I05.8	Other mitral valve diseases
I05.9	Mitral valve disease, unspecified

when of unspecified cause with mention of:

I34.-	(Nonrheumatic mitral valve disorders), code **I34.-**

I09.1	Rheumatic diseases of endocardium, valve unspecified
I09.9	Rheumatic heart disease, unspecified

with mention of:

I05-I08	(Chronic rheumatic heart disease), code **I05-I08**

I10	Essential (primary) hypertension

with mention of:

I11.-	(Hypertensive heart disease), code **I11.-**
I12.-	(Hypertensive renal disease), code **I12.-**
I13.-	(Hypertensive heart and renal disease), code **I13.-**
I20-I21	(Ischaemic heart disease), code **I20-I25**
I60-I69	(Cerebrovascular disease), code **I60-I69**
N00.-	(Acute nephritic syndrome), code **N00.-**
N01.-	(Rapidly progressive nephritic syndrome), code **N01.-**
N03.-	(Chronic nephritic syndrome), code **N03.-**
N04.-	(Nephrotic syndrome), code **N04.-**
N05.-	(Unspecified nephritic syndrome), code **N05.-**
N18.-	(Chronic renal failure), code **I12.-**
N19	(Unspecified renal failure), code **I12.-**
N26	(Unspecified contracted kidney), code **I12.-**

when reported as the originating antecedent cause of:

H35.0	(Background retinopathy and other vascular changes), code **H35.0**
I05-I09	(Conditions classifiable to I05-I09 but not specified as rheumatic), code **I34-I38**
I34-I38	(Nonrheumatic valve disorders), code **I34-I38**
I50.-	(Heart failure), code **I11.0**
I51.4-	(Complications and ill-defined
I51.9	descriptions of heart disease), code **I11.-**

I11.-   Hypertensive heart disease

with mention of:

I12.-   (Hypertensive renal disease), code **I13.-**
I13.-   (Hypertensive heart and renal disease), code **I13.-**
I20-I25   (Ischaemic heart disease), code **I20-I25**
N18.-   (Chronic renal failure), code **I13.-**
N19   (Unspecified renal failure), code **I13.-**
N26   (Unspecified contracted kidney), code **I13.-**

I12.-   Hypertensive renal disease

with mention of:

I11.-   (Hypertensive heart disease), code **I13.-**
I13.-   (Hypertensive heart and renal disease), code **I13.-**
I20-I25   (Ischaemic heart disease), code **I20-I25**

when reported as the originating antecedent cause of:

I50.-   (Heart failure), code **I13.0**
I51.4-   (Complications and ill-defined
I51.9   descriptions of heart disease), code **I13.-**

I13.-   Hypertensive heart and renal disease

with mention of:

I20-I25   (Ischaemic heart disease), code **I20-I25**

I15.-   Secondary hypertension

Not to be used for underlying cause mortality coding. If the cause is not stated, code to Other ill-defined and unspecified causes of mortality (R99).

I20.-   Angina pectoris
I24.-   Other acute ischaemic heart diseases
I25.-   Chronic ischaemic heart disease

with mention of:

I21.-   (Acute myocardial infarction), code **I21.-**
I22.-   (Subsequent myocardial infarction), code **I22.-**

I21.-   Acute myocardial infarction

with mention of:

I22.-   (Subsequent myocardial infarction), code **I22.-**

I23.-   Certain current complications following acute myocardial infarction

Not to be used for underlying cause mortality coding. Use code **I21.-** or **I22.-** as appropriate.

I24.0   Coronary thrombosis not resulting in myocardial infarction

Not to be used for underlying cause mortality coding. For mortality the occurrence of myocardial infarction is assumed and assignment made to **I21.-** or **I22.-** as appropriate

I27.9   Pulmonary heart disease, unspecified

with mention of:

M41.- (Scoliosis), code **I27.1**

I44.-   Atrioventricular and left bundle-branch block
I45.-   Other conduction disorders
I46.-   Cardiac arrest
I47.-   Paroxysmal tachycardia
I48   Atrial fibrillation and flutter
I49.-   Other cardiac arrhythmias
I50.-   Heart failure
I51.4-   Complications and ill-defined descriptions of heart
I51.9   disease

with mention of:

B57.-   (Chagas' disease), code **B57.-**
I20-I25   (Ischaemic heart diseases), code **I20-I25**

I50.-   Heart failure
I51.9   Heart disease, unspecified

with mention of:

M41.-   (Scoliosis), code **I27.1**

I50.9   Heart failure, unspecified
I51.9   Heart disease, unspecified

with mention of:

J81   (Pulmonary oedema), code **I50.1**

I65.-   Occlusion and stenosis of precerebral arteries, not resulting in cerebral infarction

I66.-   Occlusion and stenosis of cerebral arteries, not resulting in cerebral infarction

Not to be used for underlying cause mortality coding. For mortality, the occurrence of cerebral infarction is assumed and assignment made to **I63.-**.

I67.2   Cerebral atherosclerosis

with mention of:

I60-I64   (Cerebral haemorrhage, cerebral infarction or stroke), code **I60-I64**

when reported as the originating antecedent cause of conditions in:

F03 (Unspecified dementia), code **F01.-**
G20 (Parkinson's disease), code **G20**

I70.-   Atherosclerosis

with mention of:

I10-I13   (Hypertensive disease), code **I10-I13**
I20-I25   (Ischaemic heart diseases), code **I20-I25**
I51.4   (Myocarditis, unspecified), code **I51.4**
I51.5   (Myocardial degeneration), code **I51.5**
I51.6   (Cardiovascular disease, unspecified), code **I51.6**
I51.8   (Other ill-defined heart diseases), code **I51.8**
I51.9   (Heart disease, unspecified), code **I51.9**
I60-I69   (Cerebrovascular diseases), code **I60-I69**

when reported as the originating antecedent cause of:

I05-I09   (Conditions classifiable to I05-I09 but not specified as rheumatic), code **I34-I38**
I34-I38   (Nonrheumatic valve disorders), code **I34-I38**
I71-I78   (Other diseases of arteries, arterioles and capillaries), code **I71-I78**
K55.-   (Vascular disorders of intestine), code **K55.-**
N26   (Unspecified contracted kidney), code **I12.-**

I70.9   Generalized and unspecified atherosclerosis

with mention of:

R02 (Gangrene, not elsewhere classified), code **I70.2**

when reported as the originating antecedent cause of:

F03 (Unspecified dementia), code F01.-
G20 (Parkinson's disease), code **G20**

I97.-   Postprocedural disorders of circulatory system, not elsewhere classified

Not to be used for underlying cause mortality coding. See Operations, 4.2.6.

J00   Acute nasopharyngitis [common cold]
J06.-   Acute upper respiratory infections of multiple and unspecified sites

when reported as the originating antecedent cause of:

G03.8   (Meningitis), code **G03.8**
G06.0   (Intracranial abscess and granuloma), code **G06.0**
H65-H66   (Otitis media), code **H65-H66**
H70.-   (Mastoiditis and related conditions), code **H70.-**
J10-J18   (Influenza and pneumonia), code **J10-J18**
J20-J21   (Bronchitis and bronchiolitis), code **J20-J21**
J40-J42   (Unspecified and chronic bronchitis), code **J40-J42**
J44.-   (Other chronic obstructive pulmonary disease), code **J44.-**
N00.-   (Acute nephritic syndrome), code **N00.-**

J20.-   Acute bronchitis

with mention of:

J41.-   (Simple and mucopurulent chronic bronchitis), code **J41.-**
J42   (Unspecified chronic bronchitis), code **J42**
J44   (Other chronic obstructive pulmonary disease), code **J44**

J40	Bronchitis, not specified as acute or chronic
J41.-	Simple and mucopurulent chronic bronchitis
J42	Unspecified chronic bronchitis

with mention of:

J43.-	(Emphysema) code **J44.-**
J44.-	(Other chronic obstructive pulmonary disease) code **J44.-**

when reported as the originating antecedent cause of:

J45.-	(Asthma), code **J44.-** (but see also note at J45.-, J46, below)

J43.-	Emphysema

with mention of:

J40	(Bronchitis, not specified as acute or chronic), code **J44.-**
J41.-	(Simple and mucopurulent chronic bronchitis), code **J44.-**
J42	(Unspecified chronic bronchitis), code **J44.-**

J45.-	Asthma
J46	Status asthmaticus

When asthma and bronchitis (acute)(chronic) or other chronic obstructive pulmonary disease are reported together on the medical certificate of cause of death, the underlying cause should be selected by applying the General Principle or Rules 1, 2 or 3 in the normal way. Neither term should be treated as an adjectival modifier of the other.

J60-J64	Pneumoconiosis

with mention of:

A15-A16 (Respiratory tuberculosis), code **J65**

J81	Pulmonary oedema

with mention of:

I50.9	(Heart failure, unspecified), code **I50.1**
I51.9	(Heart disease, unspecified), code **I50.1**

J95.-   Postprocedural respiratory disorders, not elsewhere classified

Not to be used for underlying cause mortality coding. See Operations, 4.2.6.

K91.-   Postprocedural disorders of digestive system, not elsewhere classified

Not to be used for underlying cause mortality coding. See Operations, 4.2.6.

M41.-   Scoliosis

with mention of:

I27.9	(Pulmonary heart disease, unspecified), code **I27.1**
I50.-	(Heart failure), code **I27.1**
I51.9	(Heart disease, unspecified), code **I27.1**

M96.-   Postprocedural musculoskeletal disorders, not elsewhere classified

Not to be used for underlying cause mortality coding. See Operations, 4.2.6.

N00.-   Acute nephritic syndrome

when reported as the originating antecedent cause of:

N03.-   (Chronic nephritic syndrome), code **N03.-**

N18.-   Chronic renal failure
N19   Unspecified renal failure
N26   Unspecified contracted kidney

with mention of:

I10	(Essential (primary) hypertension), code **I12.-**
I11.-	(Hypertensive heart disease), code **I13.-**
I12.-	(Hypertensive renal disease), code **I12.-**

N46   Male infertility
N97.-   Female infertility

Not to be used if the causative condition is known.

N99.-   Postprocedural disorders of genitourinary system, not elsewhere classified

Not to be used for underlying cause mortality coding. See Operations, 4.2.6.

O08.-   Complications following abortion and ectopic and molar pregnancy

Not to be used for underlying cause mortality coding. Use categories O00-O07.

O30.-   Multiple gestation

Not to be used for underlying cause mortality coding if a more specific complication is reported.

O32.-   Maternal care for known or suspected malpresentation of fetus

with mention of :

O33.-   (Maternal care for known or suspected disproportion), code **O33.-**

O33.9   Fetopelvic disproportion

with mention of:

O33.0-O33.3   (Disproportion due to abnormality of maternal pelvis), code **O33.0-O33.3**

O64.-   Obstructed labour due to malposition and malpresentation of fetus

with mention of:

O65.-   (Obstructed labour due to maternal pelvic abnormality), code **O65.-**

O80-O84   Method of delivery

Not to be used for underlying cause mortality coding. If no other cause of maternal mortality is reported, code to Complication of labour and delivery, unspecified (O75.9)

P07.-	Disorders related to short gestation and low birth weight, not elsewhere classified
P08.-	Disorders related to long gestation and high birth weight

Not to be used if any other cause of perinatal mortality is reported.

R69.-	Unknown and unspecified causes of morbidity

Not to be used for underlying cause mortality coding. Use R95-R99 as appropriate.

S00-T98	Injury, poisoning and certain other consequences of external causes

Not to be used for underlying cause mortality coding except as an additional code to the relevant category in V01-Y89

S02.-	Fracture of skull and facial bones

When more than one site is mentioned, code to multiple fractures involving skull and facial bones, **S02.7**

S06.-	Intracranial injury

When a fracture of the skull or facial bones is associated with an intracranial injury, priority should be given to the fracture.

with mention of:

S02.-   (Fracture of skull or facial bones), code **S02.-**

T36-T50	Poisoning by drugs, medicaments and biological substances (accidental poisoning and poisoning of undetermined intent by alcohol or dependence-producing drugs)

with mention of:

F10-F19 with fourth character .2 (alcohol dependence or drug dependence), code **F10-F19** with fourth character **.2**

T79.-	Certain early complications of trauma, not elsewhere classified

Not to be used if the nature of the antecedent injury is known.

V01-X59   Accidents

with mention of:

A35   (Tetanus), code **A35**

resulting from:

G40-G41   (Epilepsy), code **G40-G41**

X40-X49   Accidental poisoning by and exposure to noxious substances
Y10-Y15   Poisoning by and exposure to noxious substances, undetermined
           intent (poisoning by alcohol or dependence-producing drugs)

with mention of:

F10-F19 with fourth character .2 (alcohol dependence or drug
dependence) code, **F10-F19** with fourth character **.2**

Y90-Y98   Supplementary factors related to causes of morbidity and
           mortality classified elsewhere

Not to be used for underlying cause mortality coding.

Z00-Z99   Factors influencing health status and contact with health services

Not to be used for underlying cause mortality coding.

4.1.12   Summary of linkages by code number

When the selected cause is listed in the first column of Table 1, and one or
more of the causes listed in the second column have been entered anywhere
on the certificate, code as indicated in the fourth column.

When the selected cause is listed in the first column and appears on the
certificate as a cause of one of the diseases listed in the third column, code as
indicated in the fourth column.

Table 1. Summary of linkages by code number

Selected cause	With mention of:	As cause of:	Resulting linked code
A00-B19 }			
B25-B99 }		C00-C97	C00-C97
A15.-, A16.-	J60-J64		J65

Selected cause	With mention of:	As cause of:	Resulting linked code
A17.-, A18.-	A15.-, A16.-		A15.-, A16.-
A39.2-A39.4	A39.0, A39.1		A39.0, A39.1
D50-D59	B20-B24		B20-B24
E86	A00-A09		A00-A09
F10-F19 (F1x.0)}	F10-F19 (F1x.2)		F10-F19 (F1x.2)
(F1x.5)}			
F10	K70.-		K70.-
F10.2	F10.4, F10.6,		F10.4, F10.6,
	F10.7		F10.7
F17.-		C34.-	C34.-
		I20-I25	I20-I25
		J40-J47	J40-J47
G25.5	I00-I02		I02.-
	I05-I09		I02.-
I05.8 }			
I05.9 }			
(of unspecified }			
cause) }	I34.-		I34.-
I09.1 }			
I09.9 }	I05-I08		I05-I08
I10	I11.-		I11.-
	I12.-		I12.-
	I13.-		I13.-
	I20-I25		I20-I25
	I60-I69		I60-I69
	N00.-		N00.-
	N01.-		N01.-
	N03-N05		N03-N05
	N18.-		I12.-
	N19		I12.-
	N26		I12.-
		H35.0	H35.0
		I05-I09	
		(not specified as	
		rheumatic)	I34-I38
		I34-I38	I34-I38
		I50.-	I11.0
		I51.4-I51.9	I11.-

Selected cause	With mention of:	As cause of:	Resulting linked code
I11.-	I12.-		I13.-
	I13.-		I13.-
	I20-I25		I20-I25
	N18.-		I13.-
	N19		I13.-
	N26		I13.-
I12.-	I11.-		I13.-
	I13.-		I13.-
	I20-I25		I20-I25
		I50.-	I13.0
		I51.4-I51.9	I13.-
I13.-	I20-I25		I20-I25
I20.- }			
I24.- }	I21.-		I21.-
I25.- }	I22.-		I22.-
I21.-	I22.-		I22.-
I27.9	M41.-		I27.1
I44-I50 }	B57.-		B57.-
I51.4-I51.9 }	I20-I25		I20-I25
I50.- }			
I51.9 }	M41.-		I27.1
I50.9 }			
I51.9 }	J81		I50.1
I67.2	I60-I64		I60-I64
		F03	F01.-
		G20	G20
I70.-	I10-I13		I10-I13
	I20-I25		I20-I25
	I51.4		I51.4
	I51.5		I51.5
	I51.6		I51.6
	I51.8		I51.8
	I51.9		I51.9
	I60-I69		I60-I69
		I05-I09 (not speficied as rheumatic)	I34-I38
		I34-I38	I34-I38
		I71-I78	I71-I78
		K55.-	K55.-
		N26	I12.-

Selected cause	With mention of:	As cause of:	Resulting linked code
I70.9	R02		I70.2
		F03	F01.-
		G20	G20
J00 }			
J06.- }		G03.8	G03.8
		G06.0	G06.0
		H65-H66	H65-H66
		H70.-	H70.-
		J10-J18	J10-J18
		J20-J21	J20-J21
		J40-J42	J40-J42
		J44.-	J44.-
		N00.-	N00.-
J20.-	J41.-		J41.-
	J42		J42
	J44.-		J44.-
J40 }			
J41.- }	J43.-		J44.-
J42 }	J44.-		J44.-
		J45.-	J44.-
J43.-	J40		J44.-
	J41.-		J44.-
	J42		J44.-
J60-J64	A15.-		J65
	A16.-		J65
J81	I50.9		I50.1
	I51.9		I50.1
M41.-	I27.9		I27.1
	I50.-		I27.1
	I51.9		I27.1
N00.-		N03.-	N03.-
N18.- }			
N19 }			
N26 }	I10		I12.-
	I11.-		I13.-
	I12.-		I12.-
O32.-	O33.-		O33.-
O33.9	O33.0-O33.3		O33.0-O33.3
O64.-	O65.-		O65.-
S06.-	S02.-		S02.-
T36-T50	F10-F19 (F1x.2)		F10-F19 (F1x.2)

Selected cause	With mention of:	As cause of:	Resulting linked code
V01-X59	A35		A35
X40-X49 }			
Y10-Y15 }	F10-F19 (F1x.2)		F10-F19 (F1x.2)

Table 2. Summary of codes not to be used in underlying cause mortality coding [a]

Codes not to be used for underlying cause mortality coding (code to item in parentheses; if no code is indicated, code to R99)		Not to be used if the underlying cause is known
B95-B97		F01-F09
E89.-		F70-F79
G97.-		G81.-
H59.-		G82.-
H95.-		G83.-
I15.-		H54.-
I23.-	(code to I21 or I22)	H90-H91
I24.0	(code to I21 or I22)	N46
I65.-	(code to I63)	N97.-
I66.-	(code to I63)	O30.-
I97.-		P07.-
J95.-		P08.-
K91.-		T79.-
M96.-		
N99.-		
O08.-		
O80-O84	(code to O75.9)	
R69.-	(code to R95-R99)	
S00-T98	(code to V01-Y89)	
Y90-Y98		
Z00-Z99		

a In addition to asterisk codes (see section 3.1.3)

4.2 Notes for interpretation of entries of causes of death

The foregoing rules will usually determine the underlying cause of death to be used for primary mortality tabulation. Each country will need to amplify the rules, depending upon the completeness and quality of medical certification. The information in this section will help in formulating such additional instructions.

4.2.1 Assumption of intervening cause

Frequently on the medical certificate, one condition is indicated as due to another, but the first one is not a direct consequence of the second one. For example, haematemesis may be stated as due to cirrhosis of the liver, instead of being reported as the final event of the sequence, liver cirrhosis→portal hypertension→ruptured oesophageal varices→haematemesis.

The assumption of an intervening cause in Part I is permissible in accepting a sequence as reported, but it must not be used to modify the coding.

Example 1:   I (a)   Cerebral haemorrhage
              (b)   Chronic nephritis

Code to chronic nephritis (N03.9). It is necessary to assume hypertension as a condition intervening between cerebral haemorrhage and the underlying cause, chronic nephritis.

Example 2:   I (a)   Mental retardation
              (b)   Premature separation of placenta

Code to premature separation of placenta affecting fetus or newborn (P02.1). It is necessary to assume birth trauma, anoxia or hypoxia as a condition intervening between mental retardation and the underlying cause, premature separation of placenta.

4.2.2 Interpretation of "highly improbable"

The expression "highly improbable" has been used since the Sixth Revision of the ICD to indicate an unacceptable causal relationship. As a guide to the acceptability of sequences in the application of the General Principle and the selection rules, the following relationships should be regarded as "highly improbable":

(a)   any infectious disease may be accepted as "due to" disorders of the immune mechanism such as human immunodeficiency virus [HIV] disease or AIDS;

(b)   an infectious or parasitic disease (A00-B99) reported as "due to" any disease outside this chapter, except that:

- diarrhoea and gastroenteritis of   )
  presumed infectious origin (A09))
- septicaemia (A40-A41)   ) may be accepted
- erysipelas (A46)   ) as "due to" any
- gas gangrene (A48.0)   ) disease
- Vincent's angina (A69.1)   )
- mycoses (B35-B49)   )
- any infectious disease may be accepted as "due to" immunosuppression by chemicals (chemotherapy) and radiation. Any infectious disease classified to A00-B19 or B25-B64 reported as "due to" a malignant neoplasm will also be an acceptable sequence.
- varicella and zoster infections (B01-B02) may be accepted as "due to" diabetes, tuberculosis and lymphoproliferative neoplasms;

(c)   a malignant neoplasm reported as "due to" any other disease, except human immunodeficiency virus [HIV] disease;

(d)   haemophilia (D66, D67, D68.0-D68.2) reported as "due to" any other disease;

(e)   diabetes (E10-E14) reported as "due to" any other disease except:
- haemochromatosis (E83.1),
- diseases of pancreas (K85-K86),
- pancreatic neoplasms (C25.-, D13.6, D13.7, D37.7),
- malnutrition (E40-E46);

(f)   rheumatic fever (I00-I02) or rheumatic heart disease (I05-I09) reported as "due to" any disease other than scarlet fever (A38), streptococcal septicaemia (A40), streptococcal sore throat (J02.0) and acute tonsillitis (J03.-);

(g)   any hypertensive condition reported as "due to" any neoplasm except:
- endocrine neoplasms,
- renal neoplasms,
- carcinoid tumours;

(h)   chronic ischaemic heart disease (I20, I25) reported as "due to" any neoplasm;

(i)   any cerebrovascular disease (I60-I69) reported as "due to" a disease of the digestive system (K00-K92) or endocarditis (I05-I08, I09.1, I33-I38), except for cerebral embolism in I65-I66 or intracranial haemorrhage (I60-I62);

(j)   any condition described as arteriosclerotic [atherosclerotic] reported as "due to" any neoplasm;

(k)   influenza (J10-J11) reported as "due to" any other disease;

(l)   a congenital anomaly (Q00-Q99) reported as "due to" any other disease of the individual, including immaturity;

(m)   a condition of stated date of onset "X" reported as "due to" a condition of stated date of onset "Y", when "X" predates "Y" (but see also Example 5 in section 4.1.6);

(n)   accidents (V01-X59) reported as due to any other cause outside this chapter except:

     (1)   any accident (V01-X59) reported as due to epilepsy (G40-G41),

     (2)   a fall (W00-W19) due to a disorder of bone density (M80-M85),

     (3)   a fall (W00-W19) due to a (pathological) fracture caused by a disorder of bone density,

     (4)   asphyxia reported as due to aspiration of mucus, blood (W80) or vomitus (W78) as a result of disease conditions,

     (5)   aspiration of food (liquid or solid) of any kind (W79) reported as due to a disease which affects the ability to swallow;

(o)   suicide (X60-X84) reported as due to any other cause.

The above list does not cover all "highly improbable" sequences, but in other cases the General Principle should be followed unless otherwise indicated.

Acute or terminal circulatory diseases reported as due to malignant neoplasm, diabetes or asthma should be accepted as possible sequences in Part I of the certificate. The following conditions are regarded as acute or terminal circulatory diseases:

I21-I22	Acute myocardial infarction
I24.-	Other acute ischaemic heart diseases
I26.-	Pulmonary embolism
I30.-	Acute pericarditis
I33.-	Acute and subacute endocarditis
I40.-	Acute myocarditis
I44.-	Atrioventricular and left bundle-branch block
I45.-	Other conduction disorders
I46.-	Cardiac arrest
I47.-	Paroxysmal tachycardia
I48	Atrial fibrillation and flutter
I49.-	Other cardiac arrhythmias
I50.-	Heart failure
I51.8	Other ill-defined heart diseases
I60-I68	Cerebrovascular diseases except I67.0-I67.5 and I67.9

4.2.3   Effect of duration on classification

In evaluating the reported sequence of the direct and antecedent causes, the interval between the onset of the disease or condition and time of death must be considered. This would apply in the interpretation of "highly improbable" relationships (see above) and in Modification Rule F (sequelae).

Categories O95 (Obstetric death of unspecified cause), O96 (Death from any obstetric cause occurring more than 42 days but less than one year after delivery) and O97 (Death from sequelae of direct obstetric causes) classify obstetric deaths according to the time elapsed between the obstetric event and the death of the woman. Category O95 is to be used when a woman dies during pregnancy, labour, delivery, or the puerperium and the only information provided is "maternal" or "obstetric" death. If the obstetric cause of death is specified, code to the appropriate category. Category O96 is used to classify deaths from direct or indirect obstetric causes that occur more than 42 days but less than a year after termination of the pregnancy. Category O97 is used to classify deaths from any direct obstetric cause which occur one year or more after termination of the pregnancy.

Conditions classified as congenital malformations, deformations and chromosomal abnormalities (Q00-Q99), even when not specified as congenital on the medical certificate, should be coded as such if the interval between onset and death and the age of the decedent indicate that the condition existed from birth.

The classification has specific categories for indicating certain diseases and injuries as the cause of sequelae or late effects. In many cases, these sequelae include conditions present one year or more after the onset of the disease or injury (see also Sequelae below).

4.2.4   Sequelae

Certain categories (B90-B94, E64.-, E68, G09, I69.-, O97 and Y85-Y89) are to be used for underlying cause mortality coding to indicate that death resulted from the late (residual) effects of a given disease or injury rather than during the active phase. Modification Rule F applies in such circumstances. Conditions reported as sequelae or residual effects of a given disease or injury should be classified to the appropriate sequela category, irrespective of the interval between the onset of the disease or injury and death. For certain conditions, deaths occurring one year or more after the onset of the disease or injury are assumed to be due to a sequela or residual effect of the condition, even though no sequela is explicitly mentioned. Guidance in interpreting sequelae is given under most of the "Sequelae of ..." categories in the tabular list.

B90.- Sequelae of tuberculosis

The sequelae include conditions specified as such or as late effects of past tuberculous disease, and residuals of tuberculosis specified as arrested, cured, healed, inactive, old, or quiescent, unless there is evidence of active tuberculosis.

B94.0 Sequelae of trachoma

The sequelae include residuals of trachoma specified as healed or inactive and certain specified sequelae such as blindness, cicatricial entropion and conjunctival scars, unless there is evidence of active infection.

B94.1 Sequelae of viral encephalitis

The sequelae include conditions specified as such, or as late effects, and those present one year or more after onset of the causal condition.

B94.8 Sequelae of other infectious and parasitic diseases

The sequelae include conditions specified as such or as late effects and residuals of these diseases described as arrested, cured, healed, inactive, old or quiescent, unless there is evidence of active disease. Sequelae also include chronic conditions reported as due to, or residual conditions present one year or more after onset of, conditions classifiable to categories A00-B89.

E64.3 Sequelae of rickets

The sequelae include any condition specified as rachitic or due to rickets and present one year or more after onset, or stated to be a sequela or late effect of rickets.

G09 Sequelae of inflammatory diseases of central nervous system

This category is provided for the coding of sequelae of conditions classifiable to G00.-, G03-G04, G06.- and G08. Sequelae of inflammatory diseases of the central nervous system subject to dual classification (G01*-G02*, G05.-* and G07*) should be coded to the categories designated for sequelae of the underlying condition (e.g. B90.0 Sequelae of central nervous system tuberculosis). If there is no sequelae category for the underlying condition, code to the underlying condition itself.

4.2.5   Consistency between sex of patient and diagnosis

Certain categories are limited to one sex (see section 3.1.5). If, after verification, the sex and cause of death on the certificate are not consistent, the death should be coded to "Other ill-defined and unspecified causes of mortality" (R99).

4.2.6   Operations

If an operation appears on the certificate as the cause of death without mention of the condition for which it was performed or of the findings at operation, and the alphabetical index does not provide a specific code for the operation, code to the residual category for the organ or site indicated by the name of the operation (e.g. code "nephrectomy" to N28.9). If the operation does not indicate an organ or site, e.g. "laparotomy", code to "Other ill-defined and unspecified causes of mortality" (R99), unless there is a mention of a therapeutic misadventure classifiable to Y60-Y84 or a postoperative complication.

4.2.7   Malignant neoplasms

When a malignant neoplasm is considered to be the underlying cause of death, it is most important to determine the primary site. Morphology and behaviour should also be taken into consideration. Cancer is a generic term and may be used for any morphological group, although it is rarely applied to malignant neoplasms of lymphatic, haematopoietic and related tissues. Carcinoma is sometimes used incorrectly as a synonym for cancer. Some death certificates may be ambiguous if there was doubt about the site of the primary or imprecision in drafting the certificate. In these circumstances, if possible, the certifier should be asked to give clarification. Failing this, the guidelines given below should be observed.

The morphological types of tumours classified in Volume 1 can be found in the Alphabetical Index with their morphology code and with an indication as to the coding by site.

A. Implication of malignancy

Mention on the certificate that a neoplasm has produced metastases (secondaries) means that it must be coded as malignant, even though this neoplasm without mention of metastases would be classified to some other section of Chapter II.

Example 1:   I (a)   Metastatic involvement of lymph nodes
             (b)   Carcinoma in situ of breast

Code to malignant neoplasm of breast (C50.9).

B. Sites with prefixes or imprecise definitions

Neoplasms of sites prefixed by "peri", "para", "pre", "supra", "infra", etc. or described as in the "area" or "region" of a site, unless these terms are specifically indexed, should be coded as follows: for morphological types classifiable to one of the categories C40, C41 (bone and articular cartilage), C43 (malignant melanoma of skin), C44 (other malignant neoplasms of skin), C45 (mesothelioma), C47 (peripheral nerves and autonomic nervous system), C49 (connective and soft tissue), C70 (meninges), C71 (brain) and C72 (other parts of central nervous system), code to the appropriate subdivision of that category; otherwise code to the appropriate subdivision of C76 (other and ill-defined sites).

Example 2:   I (a)   Fibrosarcoma in the region of the leg

Code to malignant neoplasm of connective and soft tissue of lower limb (C49.2).

C. Malignant neoplasms of unspecified site with other reported conditions

When the site of a primary malignant neoplasm is not specified, no assumption of the site should be made from the location of other reported conditions such as perforation, obstruction, or haemorrhage. These conditions may arise in sites unrelated to the neoplasm, e.g. intestinal obstruction may be caused by the spread of an ovarian malignancy.

Example 3:   I (a)   Obstruction of intestine
             (b)   Carcinoma

Code to malignant neoplasm without specification of site (C80).

D. Malignant neoplasms with primary site indicated

If a particular site is indicated as primary, it should be selected, regardless of the position on the certificate or whether in Part I or Part II. If the primary site is stated to be unknown, see E below. The primary site may be indicated in one of the following ways:

(a)   The specification of one site as primary in either Part I or II.

     Example 4:   I (a) Carcinoma of bladder
                  II   Primary in kidney

               Code to malignant neoplasm of kidney (C64).

(b)   The specification of other sites as "secondary", "metastases", "spread" or "carcinomatosis".

     Example 5:   I (a) Carcinoma of breast
                    (b) Secondaries in brain

               Code to malignant neoplasm of breast (C50.9), since Rule 2 applies

(c)   Morphology indicates a primary malignant neoplasm.

     If a morphological type implies a primary site, such as hepatoma, consider this as if the word "primary" had been included.

     Example 6:   I (a) Metastatic carcinoma
                    (b) Pseudomucinous adenocarcinoma

               Code to malignant neoplasm of ovary (C56), since pseudomucinous adenocarcinoma of unspecified site is assigned to the ovary in the Alphabetical Index.

If two or more primary sites or morphologies are indicated, these should be coded according to sections F, G and H, below.

E. Primary site unknown

If the statement, "primary site unknown", or its equivalent, appears anywhere on a certificate, code to the category for unspecified site for the morphological type involved (e.g. adenocarcinoma C80, fibrosarcoma C49.9, osteosarcoma C41.9), regardless of the site(s) mentioned elsewhere on the certificate.

     Example 7:   I (a) Secondary carcinoma of liver
                    (b) Primary site unknown
                    (c) ? Stomach ? Colon

               Code to carcinoma without specification of site (C80).

Example 8:   I (a) Generalized metastases
　　　　　　　　(b) Melanoma of back
　　　　　　　　(c) Primary site unknown

Code to malignant melanoma of unspecified site (C43.9).

F. Independent (primary) multiple sites (C97)

The presence of more than one primary neoplasm could be indicated by mention of two different anatomical sites or two distinct morphological types (e.g. hypernephroma and intraductal carcinoma), or by a mix of a morphological type that implies a specific site, plus a second site. It is highly improbable that one primary would be due to another primary malignant neoplasm except for the group of malignant neoplasms of lymphoid, haematopoietic and related tissue (C81-C96), within which one form of malignancy may terminate in another (e.g. leukaemia may follow non-Hodgkin's lymphoma).

If two or more sites mentioned in Part I are in the same organ system, see section H. If the sites are not in the same organ system and there is no indication that any is primary or secondary, code to malignant neoplasms of independent (primary) multiple sites (C97), unless all are classifiable to C81-C96, or one of the sites mentioned is a common site of metastases or the lung (see G below).

Example 9:   I (a) Cancer of stomach
　　　　　　　　 (b) Cancer of breast

Code to malignant neoplasms of independent (primary) multiple sites (C97), since two different anatomical sites are mentioned and it is unlikely that one primary malignant neoplasm would be due to another.

Example 10:   I (a) Hodgkin's disease
　　　　　　　　 (b) Carcinoma of bladder

Code to malignant neoplasms of independent (primary) multiple sites (C97), since two distinct morphological types are mentioned.

Example 11:   I (a) Acute lymphocytic leukaemia
　　　　　　　　 (b) Non-Hodgkin's lymphoma

Code to non-Hodgkin's lymphoma (C85.9), since both are classifiable to C81-C96 and the sequence is acceptable.

Example 12:   I (a) Leukaemia
              (b) Non-Hodgkin's lymphoma
              (c) Carcinoma of ovary

Code to malignant neoplasms of independent (primary) multiple sites (C97), since, although two of the neoplasms are classifiable to C81-C96, there is mention of a site elsewhere.

Example 13:   I (a) Leukaemia
              II   Carcinoma of breast

Code to leukaemia (C95.9) because the carcinoma of breast is in Part II. When dealing with multiple sites, only sites in Part I of the certificate should be considered (see H).

G. Metastatic neoplasms

When a malignant neoplasm spreads or metastasizes it generally retains the same morphology even though it may become less differentiated. Some metastases have such a characteristic microscopic appearance that the pathologist can infer the primary site with confidence, e.g. thyroid. Widespread metastasis of a carcinoma is often called carcinomatosis.If an unqualified nonspecific term such as carcinoma or sarcoma appears with a term describing a more specific histology of the same broad group, code to the site of the more specific morphology, assuming the other to be metastatic.

Although malignant cells can metastasize anywhere in the body, certain sites are more common than others and must be treated differently (see below). However, if one of these sites appears alone on a death certificate and is not qualified by the word "metastatic", it should be considered primary.

Common sites of metastases

Bone	Mediastinum
Brain	Meninges
Diaphragm	Peritoneum
Heart	Pleura
Liver	Retroperitoneum
Lung	Spinal cord
Lymph nodes	

Ill-defined sites (sites classifiable to C76)

- The lung poses special problems in that it is a common site for both metastases and primary malignant neoplasms. Lung should be considered as a common site of metastases whenever it appears with sites not on this list. However, when the bronchus or bronchogenic cancer is mentioned this neoplasm should be considered primary. If lung is mentioned and the only other sites are on the list of common sites of metastases, consider lung primary.
- Malignant neoplasm of lymph nodes not specified as primary should be assumed to be secondary.

Example 14:   I (a)   Cancer of brain

Code to malignant neoplasm of brain (C71.9).

Example 15:   I (a)   Cancer of bone
  (b)   Metastatic carcinoma of lung

Code to malignant neoplasm of lung (C34.9), since bone is on the list of common sites of metastases and lung can therefore be assumed to be primary.

The adjective "metastatic" is used in two ways - sometimes meaning a secondary from a primary elsewhere and sometimes denoting a primary that has given rise to metastases. In order to avoid confusion, the following guidelines are proposed:

(a)   **Malignant neoplasm described as "metastatic from" a specified site should be interpreted as primary of that site.**

Example 16:   I (a) Metastatic teratoma from ovary

Code to malignant neoplasm of ovary (C56).

(b)   **Malignant neoplasm described as "metastatic to" a site should be interpreted as secondary of that site unless the morphology indicates a specific primary site.**

> *Example 17:* I (a) Metastatic carcinoma to the rectum
>
> > Code to secondary malignant neoplasm of rectum (C78.5). The word "to" clearly indicates rectum as secondary.
>
> *Example 18:* I (a) Metastatic osteosarcoma to brain
>
> > Code to malignant neoplasm of bone (C41.9), since this is the unspecified site of osteosarcoma.

(c)   **A single malignant neoplasm described as "metastatic (of)".**

The terms "metastatic" and "metastatic of" should be interpreted as follows:

(i)   If one site is mentioned and this is qualified as metastatic, code to malignant primary of that particular site if no morphological type is mentioned and it is not a common metastatic site (see list of common sites of metastases given above).

> *Example 19:*   I (a) Cervical cancer, metastatic
>
> > Code to malignant neoplasm of cervix (C53.9).

(ii)   If no site is reported but the morphological type is qualified as metastatic, code as for primary site unspecified of the particular morphological type involved.

> *Example 20:*   I (a) Metastatic oat cell carcinoma
>
> > Code to malignant neoplasm of lung (C34.9).

(iii)   If a single morphological type and a site, other than a common metastatic site (see list given above), are mentioned as metastatic, code to the specific category for the morphological type and site involved.

Example 21:   I (a) Metastatic melanoma of arm

Code to malignant melanoma of skin of arm (C43.6), since in this case the ill-defined site of arm is a specific site for melanoma, not a common site of metastases classifiable to C76.

(iv)   If a single morphological type is mentioned as metastatic and the site mentioned is one of the common sites of metastases except lung, code to "unspecified site" for the morphological type, unless the unspecified site is classified to C80 (malignant neoplasm without specification of site), in which case code to secondary malignant neoplasm of the site mentioned.

Example 22:   I (a) Metastatic osteosarcoma of brain

Code to malignant neoplasm of bone, unspecified (C41.9), since brain is on the list of common sites of metastases.

(v)   If one of the common sites of metastases, except lung, is described as metastatic and no other site or morphology is mentioned, code to secondary neoplasm of the site (C77-C79).

Example 23:   I (a) Metastatic brain cancer

Code to secondary malignant neoplasm of brain (C79.3).

Example 24:   I (a) Metastatic carcinoma of lung

Code to malignant neoplasm of lung (C34.9).

(d)   More than one malignant neoplasm qualified as metastatic.

(i)   If two or more sites with the same morphology, not on the list of common sites of metastases, are reported and all are qualified as "metastatic", code as for primary site unspecified of the anatomical system and of the morphological type involved.

Example 25: I (a) Metastatic carcinoma of prostate
 (b) Metastatic carcinoma of skin

Code to malignant neoplasm without specification of site (C80), since metastatic carcinoma of prostate is not likely to be due to metastatic carcinoma of skin; both are probably due to spread from a malignant neoplasm of unknown primary site, which should have been entered on line (c).

Example 26: I (a) Metastatic carcinoma of stomach
 (b) Metastatic carcinoma of breast
 (c) Metastatic carcinoma of lung

Code to malignant neoplasm without specification of site (C80), since breast and stomach do not belong to the same anatomical system and lung is on the list of common sites of metastases.

(ii)   If two or more morphological types of different histological groups are qualified as metastatic, code to malignant neoplasms of independent (primary) multiple sites (C97) (see F).

Example 27: I (a) Bowel obstruction
 (b) Metastatic adenocarcinoma of bowel
 (c) Metastatic sarcoma of uterus

Code to malignant neoplasms of independent (primary) multiple sites (C97).

(iii) If a morphology implying site and an independent anatomical site are both qualified as metastatic, code to malignant neoplasm without specification of site (C80).

Example 28: I (a) Metastatic colonic and renal cell
 carcinoma

Code to malignant neoplasm without specification of site (C80).

(iv)   If more than one site with the same morphology is mentioned and all but one are qualified as metastatic or appear on the list of common sites of metastases, code to the site that is not qualified as metastatic, irrespective of the order of entry or whether it is in Part I or Part II. If all sites are qualified as metastatic or on the list of common sites of metastases, including lung, code to malignant neoplasm without specification of site (C80).

Example 29:   I (a) Metastatic carcinoma of stomach
    (b) Carcinoma of gallbladder
    (c) Metastatic carcinoma of colon

Code to malignant neoplasm of gallbladder (C23).

Example 30:   I (a) Metastatic carcinoma of ovary
    (b) Carcinoma of lung
    (c) Metastatic cervical carcinoma

Code to malignant neoplasm without specification of site (C80).

Example 31:   I (a) Metastatic carcinoma of stomach
    (b) Metastatic carcinoma of lung
    II   Carcinoma of colon

Code to malignant neoplasm of colon (C18.9), since this is the only diagnosis not qualified as metastatic, even though it is in Part II.

(v)   If all sites mentioned are on the list of common sites of metastases, code to unknown primary site of the morphological type involved, unless lung is mentioned, in which case code to malignant neoplasm of lung (C34.).

Example 32:   I (a) Cancer of liver
    (b) Cancer of abdomen

Code to malignant neoplasm without specification of site (C80), since both are on the list of common sites of metastases. (Abdomen is one of the ill-defined sites included in C76.-.)

Example 33:   I (a) Cancer of brain
      (b) Cancer of lung

Code to cancer of lung (C34.9), since lung in this case is considered to be primary, because brain, the only other site mentioned, is on the list of common sites of metastases.

(vi) If only one of the sites mentioned is on the list of common sites of metastases or lung, code to the site not on the list.

Example 34:   I (a) Cancer of lung
      (b) Cancer of breast

Code to malignant neoplasm of breast (C50.9), since lung in this case is considered to be a metastatic site, because breast is not on the list of common sites of metastases.

(vii) If one or more of the sites mentioned is a common site of metastases (see list given above) but two or more sites or different morphological types are also mentioned, code to malignant neoplasms of independent (primary) multiple sites (C97) (see F above).

Example 35:   I (a) Cancer of liver
      (b) Cancer of bladder
      (c) Cancer of colon

Code to malignant neoplasms of independent (primary) multiple sites (C97), since liver is on the list of common sites of metastases and there are still two other independent sites.

(viii) If there is a mixture of several sites qualified as metastatic and several other sites are mentioned, refer to the rules for multiple sites (see F above and H below).

H. Multiple sites

When dealing with multiple sites, only sites in Part I of the certificate should be considered.

If malignant neoplasms of more than one site are entered on the certificate, the site listed as primary or not indicated whether primary or secondary should be selected (see D, E and F above).

Multiple sites with none specified as primary

(a)   Notwithstanding the provisions of Rule H to consider only sites in Part I, if one of the common sites of metastases, excluding lung, and another site or morphological type are mentioned anywhere on the certificate, code to the other site. If, however, a malignant neoplasm of lymphatic, haematopoietic, or related tissue appears in Part II, only Part I should be considered.

> *Example 36:* I (a) Cancer of stomach
> (b) Cancer of liver
>
> Code to malignant neoplasm of stomach (C16.9). Although the sequence suggests that the liver was the primary site, metastasis from liver - a common site of metastases - to stomach is improbable and it is assumed that the stomach cancer metastasized to the liver.

> *Example 37:* I (a) Peritoneal cancer
> II   Mammary carcinoma
>
> Code to malignant neoplasm of breast (C50.9), since the peritoneal cancer is presumed secondary because it is on the list of common sites of metastases.

(b)   Malignant neoplasms described as one site "or" another, or if "or" is implied, should be coded to the category that embraces both sites. If no appropriate category exists, code to the unspecified site of the morphological type involved. This rule applies to all sites whether they are on the list of common sites of metastases or not.

> *Example 38:* I (a) Carcinoma of ascending or descending colon
>
> Code to malignant neoplasm of colon, unspecified (C18.9).

> *Example 39:* I (a) Osteosarcoma of lumbar vertebrae or sacrum
>
> Code to malignant neoplasm of bone, unspecified (C41.9).

(c)   If two or more morphological types of malignant neoplasm occur in lymphoid, haematopoietic or related tissue (C81-C96), code according to the sequence given since these neoplasms sometimes terminate as another entity within C81-C96. Acute exacerbation of, or blastic crisis in, chronic leukaemia should be coded to the chronic form.

Example 40: I (a) Acute lymphocytic leukaemia
                   (b) Non-Hodgkin's lymphoma

Code to non-Hodgkin's lymphoma (C85.9).

Example 41: I (a) Acute and chronic lymphocytic leukaemia

Code to chronic lymphocytic leukaemia (C91.1).

Multiple sites in the same organ system

If the sites mentioned are in the same organ system and are contiguous, the .8 subcategories, including those listed in Volume 1, should be used. This applies when the certificate describes the sites as one site "and" another or if the sites are mentioned on separate lines. Code to the .8 subcategory that embraces both sites. If there is any doubt about the contiguity of the sites mentioned, code to the unspecified site of the organ mentioned.

(a)   If there is mention of two contiguous subsites in the same site, code to the .8 subcategory of that three-character category.

Example 42: I (a) Carcinoma of descending colon and sigmoid

Code to overlapping malignant neoplasm of colon (C18.8).

(b)   If the subsites are not contiguous, code to the .9 subcategory of that three-character category.

Example 43: I (a) Carcinoma of head of pancreas
                   (b) Carcinoma of tail of pancreas

Code to malignant neoplasm of pancreas, unspecified (C25.9).

(c)   If there is mention of two contiguous sites classified to separate three-character categories within the same body system, code to the .8 subcategory of that general body system (see list in Note 5 in the introduction to Chapter II of Volume 1).

> *Example 44:* I (a) Carcinoma of vagina and cervix
>
> Code to malignant neoplasm of overlapping sites of female genital organs (C57.8).

(d)   If two sites are mentioned on the certificate and both are in the same organ system and have the same morphological type, code to the .9 subcategory of that organ system, as in the following list:

C26.9	Ill-defined sites within the digestive system
C39.9	Ill-defined sites within the respiratory system
C41.9	Bone and articular cartilage, unspecified
C49.9	Connective and soft tissue, unspecified
C57.9	Female genital organ, unspecifie
C63.9	Male genital organ, unspecified
C68.9	Urinary organ, unspecified
C72.9	Central nervous system, unspecified

> *Example 45:* I (a) Pulmonary embolism
> (b) Cancer of stomach
> (c) Cancer of gallbladder
>
> Code to ill-defined sites within the digestive system (C26.9).

(e)   If there is no available .8 or .9 subcategory, code to malignant neoplasms of independent (primary) multiple sites (C97).

> *Example 46:* I (a) Cardiac arrest
> (b) Carcinoma of prostate and bladder
>
> Code to malignant neoplasms of independent (primary) multiple sites (C97), since there is no available .8 subcategory.

I. Infectious diseases and malignant neoplasms

(a) Owing to the effect of chemotherapy on the immune system, some cancer patients become prone to infectious diseases and die of them. Therefore, any infectious disease classified to A00-B19 or B25-B64 reported as "due to" cancer will be an acceptable sequence whether in Part I or II.

> *Example 47:* I (a) Zoster
> (b) Chronic lymphocytic leukaemia
>
> Code to chronic lymphocytic leukaemia (C91.1).

(b) Except for human immunodeficiency virus [HIV] disease, no infectious or parasitic disease will be accepted as causing a malignant neoplasm.

> *Example 48:* I (a) Hepatocellular carcinoma
> (b) Hepatitis B virus
>
> Code to hepatocellular carcinoma (C22.0).

> *Example 49:* I (a) Burkitt's tumour
> (b) Epstein-Barr virus
>
> Code to Burkitt's tumour (C83.7).

> *Example 50:* I (a) Cholangiocarcinoma of liver
> (b) Clonorchiasis
>
> Code to malignant neoplasm of intrahepatic bile duct (C22.1).

J. Malignant neoplasms and circulatory disease

The following acute or fatal circulatory diseases will be accepted in Part I as due to malignant neoplasms:

> I21-I22 Acute myocardial infarction
> I24.- Other acute ischaemic heart diseases
> I26.- Pulmonary embolism
> I30.- Acute pericarditis
> I33.- Acute and subacute endocarditis
> I40.- Acute myocarditis
> I44.- Atrioventricular and left bundle-branch block
> I45.- Other conduction disorders

I46.-   Cardiac arrest
I47.-   Paroxysmal tachycardia
I48   Atrial fibrillation and flutter
I49.-   Other cardiac arrhythmias
I50.-   Heart failure
I51.8   Other ill-defined heart diseases
I60-I69 Cerebrovascular diseases, except I67.0-I67.5, I67.9, I69.-

The following circulatory diseases will not be accepted as due to malignant neoplasms:

I00-I09 Rheumatic fever and rheumatic heart disease
I10-I15 Hypertensive disease (except when reported as due to endocrine neoplasms, renal neoplasms and carcinoid tumours)
I20.-   Angina pectoris
I25.-   Chronic ischaemic heart disease
I70.-   Atherosclerosis

4.2.8   Rheumatic fever with heart involvement

If there is no statement that the rheumatic process was active at the time of death, assume activity if the heart condition (other than terminal conditions and bacterial endocarditis) that is specified as rheumatic, or stated to be due to rheumatic fever, is described as acute or subacute. In the absence of such description, the terms "carditis", "endocarditis", "heart disease", "myocarditis", and "pancarditis" can be regarded as acute if either the interval between onset and death is less than one year or, if no interval is stated, the age at death is under 15 years. "Pericarditis" can be regarded as acute at any age.

4.2.9   Congenital malformations, deformations and chromosomal abnormalities

The following conditions may be regarded as congenital when causing death at the ages stated provided there is no indication that they were acquired after birth.

- Under 1 year: aneurysm, aortic stenosis, atresia, atrophy of brain, cyst of brain, deformity, displacement of organ, ectopia, hypoplasia of organ, malformation, pulmonary stenosis, valvular heart disease.
- Under 4 weeks: heart disease NOS, hydrocephalus NOS.

If the interval between onset and death and the age of the decedent indicate that the condition existed from birth, any disease should be regarded as congenital even when not specified as congenital on the medical certificate.

4.2.10 Nature of injury

The codes for external causes (V01-Y89) should be used as the primary codes for single-condition coding and tabulation of mortality involving injury, poisoning and certain other consequences of external causes.

It is recommended that a code from Chapter XIX (S00-T98) should be used in addition in order to identify the nature of the injury and permit relevant tabulations. The following notes refer to such coding.

Where more than one kind of injury to a single body region in S00-S99, T08-T35, T66-T79 is mentioned and there is no clear indication as to which caused death, the General Principle and the Selection Rules should be applied in the normal way.

Example 1: I (a) Haemorrhagic shock
  (b) Peritoneal haemorrhage
  (c) Rupture of liver
  (d) Road traffic accident

Select rupture of liver (S36.1), since this is the starting point of the sequence terminating in the condition first entered on the certificate.

Example 2: I (a) Fat embolism
  (b) Fracture of femur
  (c) Laceration of thigh
  (d) Road traffic accident

Select fracture of femur (S72.9), since this is the starting point of the sequence terminating in the condition first entered on the certificate. It is "highly improbable" that laceration of the thigh would give rise to all the conditions mentioned above it.

Example 3: I (a) Peritonitis
  (b) Rupture of stomach and transverse colon
  (c) Road traffic accident

Select rupture of stomach (S36.3), since this is the starting point of the first-mentioned sequence (in accordance with Rule 1).

Example 4:   I (a)   Purulent meningitis
          (b)   Contusion of eyelid and penetrating wound of orbit

Select penetrating wound of orbit (S05.4), since contusion of eyelid selected by Rule 2 is obviously a direct consequence of the penetrating wound of the orbit (Rule 3 is applied).

When more than one body region is involved, coding should be made to the relevant category of Injuries involving multiple body regions (T00-T06). This applies both to the same type of injury and to more than one kind of injury to different body regions.

4.2.11   Poisoning by drugs, medicaments and biological substances

When combinations of medicinal agents classified differently are involved, proceed as follows: if one component of the combination is specified as the cause of death, code to that component; if no component is specified as the cause of death, code to the category provided for the combination, e.g. mixed antiepileptics (T42.5). Otherwise, if the components are classified to the same three-character category, code to the appropriate subcategory for "Other"; if not, code to T50.9.

Combinations of medicinal agents with alcohol should be coded to the medicinal agent.

4.2.12   External causes

The codes for external causes (V01-Y89) should be used as the primary codes for single-condition coding and tabulation of the underlying cause when, and only when, the morbid condition is classifiable to Chapter XIX (Injury, poisoning and certain other consequences of external causes).

When the morbid condition is classified to Chapters I-XVIII, the morbid condition itself should be coded as the underlying cause and categories from the chapter for external causes may be used, if desired, as supplementary codes.

4.2.13   Expressions indicating doubtful diagnosis

Qualifying expressions indicating some doubt as to the accuracy of the diagnosis, such as "apparently", "presumably", "possibly", etc., should be ignored, since entries without such qualification differ only in the degree of certainty of the diagnosis.

4.2.14   Human Immunodeficiency Virus (HIV)

When a blood transfusion is given as treatment for any condition (e.g. a haematological disorder) and an infected blood supply results in a HIV infection, code the HIV as the underlying cause and not the treated condition.

Example 1:   I (a)   Kaposi's sarcoma   1 year
        (b)   HIV   3 years
        (c)   Blood transfusion   5 years
        (d)   Haemophilia   since birth

        Code to HIV.

Example 2:   I (a)   *Pneumocystis carinii*   6 months
        (b)   HIV   5 years
        (c)   Ruptured spleen   7 years
        (d)   Assault – fist fight   7 years

        Code to HIV.

4.3   Perinatal mortality: guidelines for certification and rules for coding

4.3.1   Certification of perinatal deaths

Whenever possible, a separate certificate of cause of perinatal death should be completed, in which the causes are set out as follows:

(a)   Main disease or condition in fetus or infant
(b)   Other diseases or conditions in fetus or infant
(c)   Main maternal disease or condition affecting fetus or infant
(d)   Other maternal diseases or conditions affecting fetus or infant
(e)   Other relevant circumstances

The certificate should include identifying particulars with relevant dates and times, a statement as to whether the baby was born alive or dead, and details of the autopsy.

For a thorough analysis of perinatal mortality, the following data on both mother and child are needed, in addition to information about the causes of death, not only in the case of perinatal death, but also for all live births:

Mother
Date of birth
Number of previous pregnancies: live births/ stillbirths/ abortions
Date and outcome of last previous pregnancy: live birth/ stillbirth/abortion
Present pregnancy:
- first day of last menstrual period (if unknown, then estimated duration of pregnancy in completed weeks)
- antenatal care - two or more visits: yes/no/not known
- delivery: normal spontaneous vertex/other (specify)
Child
Birth weight in grams
Sex: boy/girl/indeterminate
Single birth/first twin/second twin/other multiple birth
If stillborn, when death occurred: before labour/during labour/not known

Other variables that might appear on the basic certificate include particulars of the birth attendant, as follows: physician/trained midwife/other trained person (specify)/other (specify).

The method by which the supplementary data are collected will vary according to the civil registration system obtaining in different countries. Where they can be collected at the registration of the stillbirth or early neonatal death, a form similar to the "Certificate of Cause of Perinatal Death" as shown below could be used. Otherwise, special arrangements would need to be made (for example, by linking birth and death records) to bring together the supplementary data and the cause of death.

Where civil registration requirements make it difficult to introduce a common death certificate for liveborn and stillborn infants, the problem could be met by separate certificates for stillbirths and early neonatal deaths, each incorporating the recommended format for the causes of death.

4.3.2   Statement of causes of death

The certificate has five sections for the entry of causes of perinatal deaths, labelled (a) to (e). In sections (a) and (b) should be entered diseases or conditions of the infant or fetus, the single most important in section (a) and the remainder, if any, in section (b). By "the single most important" is meant

the pathological condition that, in the opinion of the certifier, made the greatest contribution to the death of the infant or fetus. The mode of death, e.g. heart failure, asphyxia or anoxia, should not be entered in section (a) unless it was the only fetal or infant condition known. This also holds true for prematurity.

In sections (c) and (d) should be entered all diseases or conditions of the mother that, in the certifier's opinion, had some adverse effect on the infant or fetus. Again, the most important one of these should be entered in section (c) and the others, if any, in section (d). Section (e) is for the reporting of any other circumstances that have a bearing on the death but cannot be described as a disease or condition of the infant or mother, e.g. delivery in the absence of an attendant.

The following examples illustrate the statement of the causes of death for the cases described.

Example 1.   A woman, whose previous pregnancies had ended in spontaneous abortions at 12 and 18 weeks, was admitted when 24 weeks pregnant, in premature labour. There was spontaneous delivery of a 700 g infant who died during the first day of life. The main finding at autopsy was "pulmonary immaturity".

Causes of perinatal death:

(a) Pulmonary immaturity
(b) —
(c) Premature labour, cause unknow
(d) Recurrent aborter
(e) —

CERTIFICATE OF CAUSE OF PERINATAL DEATH

To be completed for stillbirths and liveborn infants dying within 168 hours (1 week) from birth

Identifying particulars ☐ This child was born live on   at   hours
     and died on   at   hours
     ☐ This child was stillborn on   at   hours
     and died before labour ☐   during labour ☐   not known ☐

Mother		**Child**
Date of birth ⬚⬚⬚⬚	1st day of last	Birthweight: . . . . grams
or, if unknown, age (years) ⬚	menstrual period ⬚⬚⬚⬚	Sex:
	or, if unknown, estimated duration	☐ Boy ☐ Girl ☐ Indeterminate
Number of previous	of pregnancy ⬚⬚	
pregnancies:	(completed weeks)	
Live births ⬚⬚		☐ Single birth ☐ First twin
Stillbirths ⬚⬚	Antenatal care, two or more visits:	☐ Second twin ☐ Other multiple
Abortions ⬚⬚	☐ Yes	
	☐ No	**Attendant at birth**
Outcome of last previous	☐ Not known	
pregnancy:		☐ Physician ☐ Trained midwife
☐ Live birth	Delivery:	Other trained person (specify)
☐ Stillbirth	☐ Normal spontaneous vertex	. . . .
☐ Abortion	Other (specify)	Other (specify)
Date ⬚⬚⬚⬚	. . . .	. . . .

Causes of death

a. Main disease or condition in fetus or infant

b. Other diseases or conditions in fetus or infant

c. Main maternal disease or condition affecting fetus or infant

d. Other maternal diseases or conditions affecting fetus or infant

e. Other relevant circumstances

☐ The certified cause of death has been confirmed by autopsy	I certify . . . .
	. . . .
☐ Autopsy information may be available later	. . . .
☐ Autopsy not being held	
	Signature and qualification

Example 2.   A primigravida aged 26 years with a history of regular menstrual cycles received routine antenatal care starting at the 10th week of pregnancy. At 30-32 weeks, fetal growth retardation was noted clinically, and confirmed at 34 weeks. There was no evident cause apart from symptomless bacteriuria. A caesarean section was performed and a liveborn boy weighing 1600 g was delivered. The placenta weighed 300 g and was described as infarcted. Respiratory distress syndrome developed which was responding to treatment. The baby died suddenly on the third day. Autopsy revealed extensive pulmonary hyaline membrane and massive intraventricular haemorrhage.

Causes of perinatal death:

(a) Intraventricular haemorrhage
(b) Respiratory distress syndrome
     Retarded fetal growth
(c) Placental insufficiency
(d) Bacteriuria in pregnancy
     Caesarean section

Example 3.   A known diabetic, who was poorly controlled during her first pregnancy, developed megaloblastic anaemia at 32 weeks. Labour was induced at 38 weeks. There was spontaneous delivery of an infant weighing 3200 g. The baby developed hypoglycaemia and died on the second day. Autopsy showed truncus arteriosus.

Causes of perinatal death:

(a) Truncus arteriosus
(b) Hypoglycaemia
(c) Diabetes
(d) Megaloblastic anaemia
(e) —

Example 4.   A 30-year-old mother of a healthy four-year-old boy had a
normal pregnancy apart from hydramnios. X-ray at 36 weeks
suggested anencephaly. Labour was induced. A stillborn
anencephalic fetus weighing 1500 g was delivered.

Causes of perinatal death:

(a) Anencephaly
(b) —
(c) Hydramnios
(d) —
(e) —

4.3.3   Tabulation of perinatal mortality by cause

For statistics of perinatal mortality derived from the form of certificate shown
in the accompanying documentation, full-scale multiple-cause analysis of all
conditions reported will yield the maximum benefit. Where this is
impracticable, analysis of the main disease or condition in the fetus or infant
(part (a)) and of the main maternal condition affecting the fetus or infant (part
(c)) with cross-tabulation of groups of these conditions should be regarded as
the minimum. Where it is necessary to select only one condition (for
example, when it is necessary to incorporate early neonatal deaths in single-
cause tables of deaths at all ages), the main disease or condition in the fetus
or infant (part (a)) should be selected.

4.3.4   Coding of causes of death

Each condition entered in sections (a), (b), (c) and (d) should be coded
separately. Maternal conditions affecting the infant or fetus, entered in
sections (c) and (d), should be coded to categories P00-P04 and these codes
should not be used for sections (a) and (b). Conditions in the infant or fetus,
entered in section (a), can be coded to any categories other than P00-P04 but
will most often be coded to categories P05-P96 (Perinatal conditions) or
Q00-Q99 (Congenital anomalies). Only one code should be entered for
sections (a) and (c), but for sections (b) and (d) as many codes should be
entered as there are conditions reported.

Section (e) is for review of individual perinatal deaths and will not normally
need to be coded. If, however, a statistical analysis of the circumstances
entered in section (e) is desired, some suitable categories may exist in
Chapters XX and XXI; where this is not the case, users should devise their
own coding system for this information.

4.3.5   Coding rules

The selection rules for general mortality do not apply to the perinatal death certificate. It may happen, however, that perinatal death certificates are received on which the causes of death have not been entered in accordance with the guidelines given above. Whenever possible, these certificates should be corrected by the certifier, but if this is not possible, the following rules should be applied.

Rule P1.   Mode of death or prematurity entered in section (a).

If heart or cardiac failure, asphyxia or anoxia (any condition in P20.-, P21.-) or prematurity (any condition in P07.-) is entered in section (a) and other conditions of the infant or fetus are entered in either section (a) or section (b), code the first-mentioned of these other conditions as if it had been entered alone in section (a) and code the condition actually entered in section (a) as if it had been entered in section (b).

Example 1:	Liveborn; death at 4 days	Coding
	(a) Prematurity	Q05.9
	(b) Spina bifida	P07.3
	(c) Placental insufficiency	P02.2
	(d) —	

Prematurity is coded at (b) and spina bifida at (a).

Example 2:	Liveborn; death at 50 minutes	Coding
	(a) Severe birth asphyxia	Q03.9
	Hydrocephalus	
	(b) —	P21.0
	(c) Obstructed labour	P03.1
	(d) Severe pre-eclampsia	P00.0

Severe birth asphyxia is coded at (b) and hydrocephalus at (a).

Rule P2. Two or more conditions entered in sections (a) or (c).

If two or more conditions are entered in section (a) or section (c), code the first-mentioned of these as if it had been entered alone in section (a) or (c) and code the others as if they had been entered in sections (b) or (d).

		Coding
Example 3:	Stillborn; death before onset of labour	
	(a) Severe fetal malnutrition	P05.0
	Light for dates	
	Antepartum anoxia	
	(b) —	P20.9
	(c) Severe pre-eclampsia	P00.0
	Placenta praevia	
	(d) —	P02.0

Light for dates with fetal malnutrition is coded at (a) and antepartum anoxia at (b); severe pre-eclampsia is coded at (c) and placenta praevia at (d).

		Coding
Example 4:	Liveborn; death at 2 days	
	(a) Traumatic subdural haemorrhage	P10.0
	Massive inhalation of meconium	
	Intrauterine anoxia	
	(b) Hypoglycaemia	P24.0
	Prolonged pregnancy	P20.9
		P70.4
		P08.2
	(c) Forceps delivery	P03.2
	(d) Severe pre-eclampsia	P00.0

Traumatic subdural haemorrhage is coded at (a) and the other conditions entered in (a) are coded at (b).

Rule P3. No entry in sections (a) or (c).

If there is no entry in section (a) but there are conditions of the infant or fetus entered in section (b), code the first-mentioned of these as if it had been entered in section (a); if there are no entries in either section (a) or section (b), either code P95 (Fetal death of unspecified cause) for stillbirths or code P96.9 (Condition originating in the perinatal period, unspecified) for early neonatal deaths should be used for section (a).

Similarly, if there is no entry in section (c) but there are maternal conditions entered in section (d), code the first-mentioned of these as if it had been entered in section (c); if there are no entries in either section (c) or section (d) use some artificial code, e.g. xxx.x for section (c) to indicate that no maternal condition was reported.

Example 5:	Liveborn; death at 15 minutes	Coding
	(a) —	P10.4
	(b) Tentorial tear	P22.0
	Respiratory distress syndrome	
	(c)	xxx.x
	(d) —	

Tentorial tear is coded at (a); xxx.x is coded at (c).

Example 6:	Liveborn; death at 2 days	Coding
	(a) —	P95
	(b) —	
	(c) —	P00.0
	(d) Eclampsia (longstanding essential hypertension)	

Unspecified perinatal cause is coded at (a); eclampsia is coded at (c).

Rule P4. Conditions entered in wrong section.

If a maternal condition (i.e. conditions in P00-P04) is entered in section (a) or section (b), or if a condition of the infant or fetus is entered in section (c) or section (d), code the conditions as if they had been entered in the respective correct section.

If a condition classifiable as a condition of the infant or fetus or as a maternal condition is mistakenly entered in section (e), code it as an additional fetal or maternal condition in section (b) or (d) respectively.

Example 7:   Stillborn; death after onset of labour   Coding

    (a) Severe intrauterine hypoxia   P20.9
    (b) Persistent occipitoposterior
    (c) —   P03.1
    (d) —   P03.2
    (e) Difficult forceps delivery

Persistent occipitoposterior is coded at (c); difficult forceps delivery is coded at (d).

4.4   Morbidity

At the time of the sixth revision of the ICD, adopted in 1948, a number of requests were received from public health administrators, health care managers, social security authorities and researchers in various health disciplines for a classification suitable for morbidity applications. The ICD was, therefore, made suitable for grouping morbidity data, in addition to its traditional uses, and the morbidity aspect has since been progressively expanded through successive revisions. Morbidity data are increasingly being used in the formulation of health policies and programmes, and in their management, monitoring and evaluation, in epidemiology, in identification of risk populations, and in clinical research (including studies of disease occurrence in different socioeconomic groups).

The condition to be used for single-condition morbidity analysis is the main condition treated or investigated during the relevant episode of health care. The main condition is defined as the condition, diagnosed at the end of the episode of health care, primarily responsible for the patient's need for treatment or investigation. If there is more than one such condition, the one held most responsible for the greatest use of resources should be selected. If no diagnosis was made, the main symptom, abnormal finding or problem should be selected as the main condition.

In addition to the main condition, the record should, whenever possible, also list separately other conditions or problems dealt with during the episode of health care. Other conditions are defined as those conditions that coexist or develop during the episode of health care and affect the management of the patient. Conditions related to an earlier episode that have no bearing on the current episode should not be recorded.

By limiting analysis to a single condition for each episode, some available information may be lost. It is therefore recommended, where practicable, to carry out multiple-condition coding and analysis to supplement the routine data. This should be done according to local rules, since no international rules have been established. However, experience in other areas could be useful in developing local schemes.

4.4.1 Guidelines for recording diagnostic information for single-condition analysis of morbidity data

General

The health care practitioner responsible for the patient's treatment should select the main condition to be recorded, as well as any other conditions, for each episode of health care. This information should be organized systematically by using standard recording methods. A properly completed record is essential for good patient management and is a valuable source of epidemiological and other statistical data on morbidity and other health care problems.

Specificity and detail

Each diagnostic statement should be as informative as possible in order to classify the condition to the most specific ICD category. Examples of such diagnostic statements include:

- transitional cell carcinoma of trigone of bladder
- acute appendicitis with perforation
- diabetic cataract, insulin-dependent
- meningococcal pericarditis
- antenatal care for pregnancy-induced hypertension
- diplopia due to allergic reaction to antihistamine taken as prescribed
- osteoarthritis of hip due to an old hip fracture
- fracture of neck of femur following a fall at home
- third-degree burn of palm of hand.

Uncertain diagnoses or symptoms

If no definite diagnosis has been established by the end of an episode of health care, then the information that permits the greatest degree of specificity and knowledge about the condition that necessitated care or investigation should be recorded. This should be done by stating a symptom, abnormal finding or problem, rather than qualifying a diagnosis as "possible", "questionable" or "suspected", when it has been considered but not established.

Contact with health services for reasons other than illness

Episodes of health care or contact with health services are not restricted to the treatment or investigation of current illness or injury. Episodes may also occur when someone who may not currently be sick requires or receives limited care or services; the details of the relevant circumstances should be recorded as the "main condition". Examples include:

- monitoring of previously treated conditions
- immunization
- contraceptive management, antenatal and postpartum care
- surveillance of persons at risk because of personal or family history
- examinations of healthy persons, e.g. for insurance or occupational reasons
- seeking of health-related advice
- requests for advice by persons with social problems
- consultation on behalf of a third party.

Chapter XXI (Factors influencing health status and contact with health services) provides a broad range of categories (Z00-Z99) for classifying these circumstances; reference to this chapter will give an indication of the detail required to permit classification to the most relevant category.

Multiple conditions

Where an episode of health care concerns a number of related conditions (e.g. multiple injuries, multiple sequelae of a previous illness or injury, or multiple conditions occurring in human immunodeficiency virus [HIV] disease), the one that is clearly more severe and demanding of resources than the others should be recorded as the "main condition" and the others as "other conditions". Where no one condition predominates, a term such as "multiple fractures", "multiple head injuries", or "HIV disease resulting in multiple infections" may be recorded as the "main condition", followed by a list of the conditions. If there are a number of such conditions, with none predominating, then a term such as "multiple injuries" or "multiple crushing injuries" should be recorded alone.

Conditions due to external causes

When a condition such as an injury, poisoning or other effect of external causes is recorded, it is important to describe fully both the nature of the condition and the circumstances that gave rise to it. For example: "fracture of neck of femur caused by fall due to slipping on greasy pavement"; "cerebral contusion caused when patient lost control of car, which hit a tree"; "accidental poisoning - patient drank disinfectant in mistake for soft drink"; or "severe hypothermia - patient fell in her garden in cold weather".

Treatment of sequelae

Where an episode of care is for the treatment or investigation of a residual condition (sequela) of a disease that is no longer present, the sequela should be fully described and its origin stated, together with a clear indication that the original disease is no longer present. For example: "deflected nasal septum - fracture of nose in childhood", "contracture of Achilles tendon - late effect of injury to tendon", or "infertility due to tubal occlusion from old tuberculosis".

Where multiple sequelae are present and treatment or investigation is not directed predominantly at one of them, a statement such as "sequelae of cerebrovascular accident" or "sequelae of multiple fractures" is acceptable.

4.4.2 Guidelines for coding "main condition" and "other conditions"

General

The "main condition" and "other conditions" relevant to an episode of health care should have been recorded by the responsible health care practitioner, and coding is therefore usually straightforward, since the main condition stated should be accepted for coding and processing unless it is obvious that the guidelines given above have not been followed. Whenever possible, a record with an obviously inconsistent or incorrectly recorded main condition should be returned for clarification. Failing clarification, Rules MB1 to MB5 (section 4.4.3) will help the coder to deal with some of the commoner causes of incorrect recording. The guidelines given below are for use when the coder may be unclear as to which code should be used.

It has been recommended that "other conditions" in relation to an episode of care should be recorded in addition to the main condition, even for single-cause analysis, since this information may assist in choosing the correct ICD code for the main condition.

Optional additional codes

In the guidelines below, a preferred code for the "main condition" is sometimes indicated, together with an optional additional code to give more information. The preferred code indicates the "main condition" for single-cause analysis and an additional code may be included for multiple-cause analysis.

Coding of conditions to which the dagger and asterisk system applies

If applicable, both dagger and asterisk codes should be used for the main condition, since they denote two different pathways for a single condition.

Example 1: Main condition: Measles pneumonia
Other conditions: —

Code to measles complicated by pneumonia (B05.2†) and pneumonia in viral diseases classified elsewhere (J17.1*).

Example 2: Main condition: Tuberculous pericarditis
Other conditions: —

Code to tuberculosis of other specified organs (A18.8†) and pericarditis in bacterial diseases classified elsewhere (I32.0*).

Example 3: Main condition: Lyme disease arthritis
Other conditions: —

Code to Lyme disease (A69.2†) and arthritis in Lyme disease (M01.2*).

Coding of suspected conditions, symptoms and abnormal findings and non-illness situations

If the period of health care was for an inpatient, the coder should be cautious about classifying the main condition to Chapters XVIII and XXI. If a more specific diagnosis has not been made by the end of the inpatient stay, or if there was truly no codable current illness or injury, then codes from the above chapters are permissible (see also Rules MB3 and MB5, section 4.4.3). The categories can be used in the normal way for other episodes of contact with health services.

If, after an episode of health care, the main condition is still recorded as "suspected", "questionable", etc., and there is no further information or clarification, the suspected diagnosis must be coded as if established.

Category Z03.- (Medical observation and evaluation for suspected diseases and conditions) applies to suspected diagnoses that can be ruled out after investigation.

Example 4: Main condition: Suspected acute cholecystitis
Other conditions: —

Code to acute cholecystitis (K81.0) as "main condition".

Example 5:   Main condition: Admitted for investigation of suspected malignant neoplasm of cervix - ruled out

Code to observation for suspected malignant neoplasm (Z03.1) as "main condition".

Example 6:   Main condition: Ruled out myocardial infarction
Other conditions: —

Code to observation for suspected myocardial infarction (Z03.4) as "main condition".

Example 7:   Main condition: Severe epistaxis
Other conditions: —

Patient in hospital one day. No procedures or investigations reported

Code to epistaxis (R04.0). This is acceptable since the patient was obviously admitted to deal with the immediate emergency only.

Coding of multiple conditions

Where multiple conditions are recorded in a category entitled "Multiple ...", and no single condition predominates, the code for the "Multiple ..." category should be used as the preferred code, and optional additional codes may be added for individual conditions listed.

Such coding applies mainly to conditions associated with HIV disease, to injuries and sequelae.

Coding of combination categories

The ICD provides certain categories where two conditions or a condition and an associated secondary process can be represented by a single code. Such combination categories should be used as the main condition where appropriate information is recorded. The Alphabetical Index indicates where such combinations are provided for, under the indent "with", which appears immediately after the lead term. Two or more conditions recorded under "main condition" may be linked if one of them may be regarded as an adjectival modifier of the other.

Example 8:   Main condition: Renal failure
Other conditions: Hypertensive renal disease

Code to hypertensive renal disease with renal failure (I12.0) as the "main condition".

Example 9:   Main condition: Glaucoma secondary to eye
                                   inflammation
                Other conditions: —

Code to glaucoma secondary to eye inflammation (H40.4) as the "main condition".

Example 10:   Main condition: Intestinal obstruction
                Other conditions: Left inguinal hernia

Code to unilateral or unspecified inguinal hernia, with obstruction, without gangrene (K40.3).

Example 11:   Main condition: Cataract. Insulin-dependent diabetes
                Other conditions: Hypertension
                Specialty: Ophthalmology

Code to insulin-dependent diabetes with ophthalmic complications (E10.3†) and diabetic cataract (H28.0*) as the "main condition".

Example 12:   Main condition: Non-insulin-dependent diabetes
                                   mellitus
                Other conditions: Hypertension
                                   Rheumatoid arthritis
                                   Cataract
                Specialty: General medicine

Code to non-insulin-dependent diabetes without complications (E11.9) as "main condition". Note that in this example the linkage of cataract with diabetes must not be made since they are not both recorded under "main condition".

Coding of external causes of morbidity

For injuries and other conditions due to external causes, both the nature of the condition and the circumstances of the external cause should be coded. The preferred "main condition" code should be that describing the nature of the condition. This will usually, but not always, be classifiable to Chapter XIX. The code from Chapter XX indicating the external cause would be used as an optional additional code.

Example 13:   Main condition: Fracture of neck of femur caused by
                                   fall due to tripping on uneven
                                   pavement
                Other conditions: Contusions to elbow and upper arm

Code to fracture of neck of femur (S72.0) as "main condition". The external cause code for fall on same level from slipping, tripping or stumbling on street or highway (W01.4) may be used as an optional additional code.

Example 14:   Main condition: Severe hypothermia - patient fell in
                                      her garden in cold weather
               Other conditions: Senility

Code to hypothermia (T68) as "main condition". The external cause code for exposure to excessive natural cold at home (X31.0) may be used as an optional additional code.

Example 15:   Main condition: Diplopia due to allergic reaction to
                                      antihistamine taken as prescribed
               Other conditions: —

Code to diplopia (H53.2) as the "main condition". The external cause code for antiallergic and antiemetic drugs causing adverse effects in therapeutic use (Y43.0) may be used as an optional additional code.

Example 16:   Main condition: Haemoglobinuria caused by training
                                      for marathon run (training on outdoor
                                      track at stadium)
               Other conditions: —

Code to haemoglobinuria due to haemolysis from other external causes (D59.6) as "main condition". The external cause code for overexertion and strenuous, repetitive movements at sports and athletics area (X50.3) may be used as an optional additional code.

Coding of sequelae of certain conditions

The ICD provides a number of categories entitled "Sequelae of ..." (B90-B94, E64.-, E68, G09, I69.-, O97, T90-T98, Y85-Y89) which may be used to indicate conditions no longer present as the cause of a current problem undergoing treatment or investigation. The preferred code for the "main condition" is, however, the code for the nature of the sequela itself, to which the code for "Sequelae of ..." may be added as an optional additional code.

Where a number of different very specific sequelae are present and no one of them predominates in severity and use of resources for treatment, it is permissible for the description "Sequelae of ..." to be recorded as the "main condition" and this may then be coded to the appropriate category. Note that it is sufficient that the causal condition is described as "old", "no longer present", etc. or the resulting condition is described as "late effect of ...", or "sequela of ..." for this to apply. There is no minimum time interval.

Example 17: Main condition: Dysphasia from old cerebral infarction
Other conditions: —

Code to dysphasia (R47.0) as the "main condition". The code for sequelae of cerebral infarction (I69.3) may be used as an optional additional code.

Example 18: Main condition: Osteoarthritis of hip joint due to old hip fracture from motor vehicle accident 10 years ago
Other conditions: —

Code to other post-traumatic coxarthrosis (M16.5) as the "main condition". The codes for sequelae of fracture of femur (T93.1) and sequelae of motor vehicle accident (Y85.0) may be used as optional additional codes.

Example 19: Main condition: Late effects of poliomyelitis
Other conditions: —

Code to sequelae of poliomyelitis (B91) as the "main condition" since no other information is available.

Coding of acute and chronic conditions

Where the main condition is recorded as being both acute (or subacute) and chronic, and the ICD provides separate categories or subcategories for each, but not for the combination, the category for the acute condition should be used as the preferred main condition.

Example 20: Main condition: Acute and chronic cholecystitis
Other conditions: —

Code to acute cholecystitis (K81.0) as the "main condition". The code for chronic cholecystitis (K81.1) may be used as an optional additional code.

Example 21: Main condition: Acute exacerbation of chronic obstructive bronchitis
Other conditions: —

Code to chronic obstructive pulmonary disease with acute exacerbation (J44.1) as the "main condition" since the ICD provides an appropriate code for the combination.

Coding of postprocedural conditions and complications

Categories are provided in Chapter XIX (T80-T88) for certain complications related to surgical and other procedures, e.g. surgical wound infections, mechanical complications of implanted devices, shock, etc. Most body-system chapters also contain categories for conditions that occur either as a consequence of specific procedures and techniques or as a result of the removal of an organ, e.g. postmastectomy lymphoedema syndrome, post-irradiation hypothyroidism. Some conditions (e.g. pneumonia, pulmonary embolism) that may arise in the postprocedural period are not considered unique entities and are, therefore, coded in the usual way, but an optional additional code from Y83-Y84 may be added to identify the relationship to a procedure.

When postprocedural conditions and complications are recorded as the main condition, reference to modifiers or qualifiers in the Alphabetical Index is essential for choosing the correct code.

Example 22: Main condition: Hypothyroidism since thyroidectomy 1 year ago

Other conditions: —
Specialty: General medicine

Code to postsurgical hypothyroidism (E89.0) as the "main condition".

Example 23: Main condition: Excessive haemorrhage after tooth extraction

Other conditions: Pain
Specialty: Dentistry

Code to haemorrhage resulting from a procedure (T81.0) as the "main condition".

Example 24: Main condition: Postoperative psychosis after plastic surgery

Other conditions: —
Specialty: Psychiatry

Code to psychosis (F09) as the "main condition" and supplement by Y83.8 (other specified surgical procedures [as the cause of abnormal reaction of the patient]) to indicate the postprocedural relationship.

4.4.3   Rules for reselection when the main condition is incorrectly recorded

The responsible health care practitioner indicates the "main condition" to be coded, and this should normally be accepted for coding subject to the guidelines above and in the chapter-specific notes in section 4.4.4. However, certain circumstances or the availability of other information may indicate that the health care practitioner has not followed the correct procedure. If it is not possible to obtain clarification from the health care practitioner, one of the following rules may be applied and the "main condition" reselected.

Rules for reselection of main condition

Rule MB1.   *Minor condition recorded as "main condition", more significant condition recorded as "other condition"*

Where a minor or longstanding condition, or an incidental problem, is recorded as the "main condition", and a more significant condition, relevant to the treatment given and/or the specialty that cared for the patient, is recorded as an "other condition", reselect the latter as the "main condition".

Rule MB2.   *Several conditions recorded as "main condition".*

If several conditions that cannot be coded together are recorded as the "main condition", and other details on the record point to one of them as the "main condition" for which the patient received care, select that condition. Otherwise select the condition first mentioned.

Rule MB3.   *Condition recorded as "main condition" is presenting symptom of diagnosed, treated condition*

If a symptom or sign (usually classifiable to Chapter XVIII), or a problem classifiable to Chapter XXI, is recorded as the "main condition" and this is obviously the presenting sign, symptom or problem of a diagnosed condition recorded elsewhere and care was given for the latter, reselect the diagnosed condition as the "main condition".

Rule MB4.   *Specificity*

Where the diagnosis recorded as the "main condition" describes a condition in general terms, and a term that provides more precise information about the site or nature of the condition is recorded elsewhere, reselect the latter as the "main condition".

Rule MB5.   Alternative main diagnoses

Where a symptom or sign is recorded as the "main condition" with an indication that it may be due to either one condition or another, select the symptom as the "main condition". Where two or more conditions are recorded as diagnostic options for the "main condition", select the first condition recorded.

Examples of application of the rules for reselection of main condition

Rule MB1.   Minor condition recorded as "main condition", more significant condition recorded as "other condition"

Where a minor or longstanding condition, or an incidental problem, is recorded as the "main condition", and a more significant condition, relevant to the treatment given and/or the specialty that cared for the patient, is recorded as an "other condition", reselect the latter as the "main condition".

Example 1:	Main condition:	Acute sinusitis
	Other conditions:	Carcinoma of endocervix
		Hypertension
		Patient in hospital for three weeks
	Procedure:	Total hysterectomy
	Specialty:	Gynaecology

Reselect carcinoma of endocervix as the "main condition" and code to C53.0.

Example 2:	Main condition:	Rheumatoid arthritis
	Other conditions:	Diabetes mellitus
		Strangulated femoral hernia
		Generalized arteriosclerosis
		Patient in hospital for two weeks
	Procedure:	Herniorrhaphy
	Specialty:	Surgery

Reselect strangulated femoral hernia as the "main condition" and code to K41.3.

Example 3:	Main condition:	Epilepsy
	Other conditions:	Otomycosis
	Specialty:	Ear, nose and throat

Reselect otomycosis as the "main condition" and code to B36.9† and H62.2*.

Example 4:	Main condition:	Congestive heart failure
	Other conditions: bed during	Fracture neck of femur due to fall from hospitalization
		Patient in hospital for four weeks
	Procedure:	Internal fixation of fracture
	Specialty:	Internal medicine for 1 week then transfer to orthopaedic surgery for treatment of fracture

Reselect fracture of neck of femur as the "main condition" and code to S72.0.

Example 5:	Main condition:	Dental caries
	Other conditions:	Rheumatic mitral stenosis
	Procedure:	Dental extractions
	Specialty:	Dentistry

Select dental caries as the "main condition" and code to K02.9. Rule MB1 does not apply. Although dental caries can be regarded as a minor condition and rheumatic mitral stenosis as a more significant condition, the latter was not the condition treated during the episode of care.

Rule MB2.   Several conditions recorded as "main condition"

If several conditions that cannot be coded together are recorded as the "main condition", and other details on the record point to one of them as being the "main condition" for which the patient received care, select that condition. Otherwise select the condition first mentioned.

Note: See also 4.4.2, coding of multiple conditions and coding of combination categories.

Example 6:	Main condition:	Cataract
		Staphylococcal meningitis
		Ischaemic heart disease
	Other conditions:	—
		Patient in hospital for five weeks
	Specialty:	Neurology

Select staphylococcal meningitis as the "main condition" and code to G00.3.

Example 7: Main condition: Chronic obstructive bronchitis
                                Hypertrophy of prostate
                                Psoriasis vulgaris

Outpatient in the care of a dermatologist

Select psoriasis vulgaris as the "main condition" and code to L40.0.

Example 8: Main condition: Mitral stenosis
                                Acute bronchitis
                                Rheumatoid arthritis
              Other conditions: —
              Specialty: General medicine
              No information about therapy

Select mitral stenosis, the first-mentioned condition, as the "main condition" and code to I05.0.

Example 9: Main condition: Chronic gastritis
                                Secondary malignancy in axillary
                                lymph nodes
                                Carcinoma of breast
              Other conditions: —
              Procedure: Mastectomy

Select malignant neoplasm of breast as the "main condition" and code to C50.9.

Example 10: Main condition: Premature rupture of membranes
                                Breech presentation
                                Anaemia
              Other conditions: —
              Procedure: Spontaneous delivery

Select premature rupture of membranes, the first-mentioned condition, as the "main condition" and code to O42.9.

Rule MB3.   Condition recorded as "main condition" is presenting symptom of diagnosed, treated condition

If a symptom or sign (usually classifiable to Chapter XVIII), or a problem classifiable to Chapter XXI, is recorded as the "main condition" and this is obviously the presenting sign, symptom or problem of a diagnosed condition recorded elsewhere and care was given for the latter, reselect the diagnosed condition as the "main condition".

Example 11:	Main condition:	Haematuria
	Other conditions:	Varicose veins of legs
		Papillomata of posterior wall of bladder
	Treatment:	Diathermy excision of papillomata
	Specialty:	Urology

Reselect papillomata of posterior wall of bladder as the "main condition" and code to D41.4.

Example 12:	Main condition:	Coma
	Other conditions:	Ischaemic heart disease
		Otosclerosis
		Diabetes mellitus, insulin-dependent
	Specialty:	Endocrinology
	Care:	Establishment of correct dose of insulin

Reselect diabetes mellitus, insulin-dependent as the "main condition" and code to E10.0. The information provided indicates that the coma was due to diabetes mellitus and coma is taken into account as it modifies the coding.

Example 13:	Main condition:	Abdominal pain
	Other conditions:	Acute appendicitis
	Procedure:	Appendectomy

Reselect acute appendicitis as the "main condition" and code to K35.9.

Example 14:	Main condition:	Febrile convulsions
	Other conditions:	Anaemia

No information about therapy

Accept febrile convulsions as the "main condition" and code to R56.0. Rule MB3 does not apply since the "main condition" as reported is not a presenting symptom of the other reported condition.

Rule MB4.   Specificity

Where the diagnosis recorded as the "main condition" describes a condition in general terms, and a term that provides more precise information about the site or nature of the condition is recorded elsewhere, reselect the latter as the "main condition".

Example 15: Main condition: Cerebrovascular accident
              Other conditions: Diabetes mellitus
                                 Hypertension
                                 Cerebral haemorrhage

Reselect cerebral haemorrhage as the "main condition" and code to I61.9.

Example 16: Main condition: Congenital heart disease
              Other conditions: Ventricular septal defect

Reselect ventricular septal defect as the "main condition" and code to Q21.0.

Example 17: Main condition: Enteritis
              Other conditions: Crohn's disease of ileum

Reselect Crohn's disease of ileum as the "main condition" and code to K50.0.

Example 18: Main condition: Dystocia
              Other conditions: Hydrocephalic fetus
                                 Fetal distress
              Procedure: Caesarean section

Reselect obstructed labour due to other abnormalities of fetus as the "main condition" and code to O66.3.

Rule MB5.   *Alternative main diagnoses*

Where a symptom or sign is recorded as the "main condition" with an indication that it may be due to either one condition or another, select the symptom as the "main condition". Where two or more conditions are recorded as diagnostic options for the "main condition", select the first condition recorded.

Example 19: Main condition: Headache due to either stress and
                               tension or acute sinusitis
              Other conditions: —

Select headache as the "main condition" and code to R51.

Example 20: Main condition: Acute cholecystitis or acute
                               pancreatitis
              Other conditions: —

Select acute cholecystitis as the "main condition" and code to K81.0.

Example 21:   Main condition: Gastroenteritis due to infection or food poisoning

Other conditions: —

Select infectious gastroenteritis as the "main condition" and code to A09.

4.4.4   Chapter-specific notes

Guidance is given below for specific chapters where problems may be encountered in selecting preferred "main condition" codes. The preceding general guidelines and rules apply to all chapters unless a specific chapter note states otherwise.

Chapter I: Certain infectious and parasitic diseases

B20-B24 Human immunodeficiency virus [HIV] disease

A patient with a compromised immune system due to HIV disease may sometimes require treatment during the same episode of care for more than one disease, for example mycobacterial and cytomegalovirus infections. Categories and subcategories are provided in this block for HIV disease with various other resultant diseases. Code the appropriate subcategory for the "main condition" as selected by the health care practitioner.

Where the "main condition" has been recorded as HIV disease with multiple accompanying diseases, the appropriate .7 subcategory from B20-B22 should be coded. Conditions classifiable to two or more subcategories of the same category should be coded to the .7 subcategory of the relevant category (e.g. B20 or B21). Subcategory B22.7 should be used when conditions classifiable to two or more categories from B20-B22 are present. Additional codes from within the block B20-B24 may be used, if desired, to specify the individual conditions listed.

In those rare instances when the associated condition clearly predates the HIV infection, the combination should not be coded and the selection rules should be followed.

Example 1:   Main condition: HIV disease and Kaposi's sarcoma
Other conditions: —

Code to HIV disease resulting in Kaposi's sarcoma (B21.0).

Example 2:   Main condition: Toxoplasmosis and cryptococcosis in HIV patient

Other conditions: —

> Code to HIV disease resulting in multiple infections (B20.7). B20.8 (HIV disease resulting in other infectious and parasitic diseases) and B20.5 (HIV disease resulting in other mycoses) may be used as additional codes, if desired.

Example 3:   Main condition: HIV disease with *Pneumocystis carinii* pneumonia, Burkitt's lymphoma and oral candidiasis

Other conditions: —

> Code to HIV disease resulting in multiple diseases (B22.7). Additional codes B20.6 (HIV disease resulting in *Pneumocystis carinii* pneumonia), B21.1 (HIV disease resulting in Burkitt's lymphoma) and B20.4 (HIV disease resulting in candidiasis) may be used, if desired.

The subcategories at B20-B23 are the only optional four-character codes for countries using the four-character version of ICD-10. Where it is not desired to use these optional fourth-character subcategories, codes from elsewhere in the classification should be used as additional codes to identify the specific resultant conditions. In Example 1 above, the "main condition" would be coded to B21 (HIV disease resulting in malignant neoplasm). Code C46.9 (Kaposi's sarcoma) would be used as an additional code. In Example 2, the "main condition" would be coded to B20 (HIV disease resulting in infectious and parasitic diseases). Codes B58.9 (Toxoplasmosis, unspecified) and B45.9 (Cryptococcosis, unspecified) would be used as additional codes.

Whether to use the four-character subcategories of B20-B23 or multiple-cause coding to identify the specific conditions is a policy decision which should be made at the time ICD-10 is implemented.

B90-B94 Sequelae of infectious and parasitic diseases

These codes are not to be used as the preferred codes for "main condition" if the nature of the residual condition is recorded. When coding to the residual condition, B90-B94 may be used as optional additional codes (see 4.4.2, Coding of sequelae of certain conditions).

B95-B97 Bacterial, viral and other infectious agents

These codes are not to be used as "main condition" codes. The categories are provided for optional use as additional codes to identify the infectious agent or organism in diseases classified outside Chapter I. Infections of unspecified site due to these agents are classified elsewhere in Chapter I.

Example 4:   Main condition: Acute cystitis due to *E. coli*
                    Other conditions: —

Code to acute cystitis (N30.0) as the "main condition", B96.2 (*E. coli* as the cause of diseases classified to other chapters) may be used as an optional additional code.

Example 5:   Main condition: Bacterial infection
                    Other conditions: —

Code to bacterial infection, unspecified (A49.9), as the "main condition", not to a code from B95-B97.

Chapter II: Neoplasms

When coding neoplasms, refer to the notes introducing Chapter II in Volume 1 and to the introduction of the Alphabetical Index (Volume 3) regarding code assignment and the use of morphological descriptions.

A neoplasm, whether primary or metastatic, that is the focus of care during a relevant episode of health care, should be recorded and coded as the "main condition". When the "main condition" as recorded by the health care practitioner is a primary neoplasm that is no longer present (having been removed during a previous episode of care), code as the "main condition" the neoplasm of the secondary site, the current complication, or the appropriate circumstance codable to Chapter XXI (see 4.4.1, Contact with health services for reasons other than illness) that was the focus of the treatment or investigation during the current episode of care. An appropriate code from Chapter XXI for personal history of neoplasm may be used as an optional additional code.

Example 6:   Main condition: Carcinoma of prostate
                    Other conditions: Chronic bronchitis
                    Procedure: Prostatectomy

Code to malignant neoplasm of prostate (C61) as the "main condition".

Example 7:   Main condition: Carcinoma of breast - resected two years ago
                    Other conditions: Secondary carcinoma in lung
                    Procedure: Bronchoscopy with biopsy

Code to secondary malignant neoplasm of lung (C78.0) as the "main condition". Z85.3 (Personal history of malignant neoplasm of breast) may be used as an optional additional code.

Example 8:   Main condition: Previously excised bladder cancer -
                                    admitted for follow-up examination by
                                    cystoscopy
                Other conditions: —
                Procedure: Cystoscopy

Code to follow-up examination after surgery for malignant neoplasm (Z08.0) as the "main condition". Z85.5 (Personal history of malignant neoplasm of urinary tract) may be used as an optional additional code.

C80   Malignant neoplasm without specification of site

C97   Malignant neoplasms of independent (*primary*) multiple sites

C80 should be used for "main condition" coding only when the health care practitioner has clearly recorded the neoplasm in such a manner. C97 should be used when the health care practitioner records as the "main condition" two or more independent primary malignant neoplasms, none of which predominates. Additional codes may be used to identify the individual malignant neoplasms listed.

Example 9:   Main condition: Carcinomatosis
                Other conditions: —

Code to malignant neoplasm without specification of site (C80).

Example 10: Main condition: Multiple myeloma and primary
                                    adenocarcinoma of prostate
                Code to malignant neoplasms of independent (primary) multiple sites (C97). C90.0 (Multiple myeloma) and C61 (Malignant neoplasm of prostate) may be used as optional additional codes.

Chapter III: Diseases of the blood and blood-forming organs and certain disorders involving the immune mechanism

Certain conditions classifiable to this chapter may result from drugs or other external causes. Codes from Chapter XX may be used as optional additional codes.

Example 11:   Main condition: Trimethoprim-induced folate
                                                   deficiency anaemia
               Other conditions: —

               Code drug-induced folate deficiency anaemia (D52.1) as the
               "main condition". Y41.2 (Antimalarials and drugs acting on
               other blood protozoa causing adverse effects in therapeutic
               use) may be used as an optional additional code.

Chapter IV: Endocrine, nutritional and metabolic diseases

Certain conditions classifiable to this chapter may result from drugs or other
external causes. Codes from Chapter XX may be used as optional additional
codes.

E10-E14 Diabetes mellitus

In coding the "main condition", the selection of an appropriate subcategory
from the list that applies to all of these categories should be based on the
"main condition" as recorded by the health care practitioner. The subcategory
.7 should be used as the "main condition" code only when multiple
complications of diabetes have been recorded as the "main condition"
without preference for any one complication. Codes for any individual
complications listed may be added as optional additional codes.

Example 12:   Main condition: Renal failure due to diabetic
                                                   glomerulonephrosis
               Code   to   unspecified   diabetes   mellitus   with   renal
               complications (E14.2† and N08.3*).

Example 13:   Main condition: Insulin-dependent diabetic with
                                                   nephropathy, gangrene and cataracts
               Other conditions: —

               Code to insulin-dependent diabetes mellitus with multiple
               complications (E10.7). Codes E10.2† and N08.3* (Insulin-
               dependent diabetes with nephropathy), E10.5 (Insulin-
               dependent   diabetes   with   peripheral   circulatory
               complications) and E10.3† and H28.0* (Insulin-dependent
               diabetes with cataract) may be added as optional additional
               codes to identify the individual complications.

E34.0 Carcinoid syndrome

This code is not to be used as the preferred code for the "main condition" if a carcinoid tumour is recorded, unless the episode of care was directed predominantly at the endocrine syndrome itself. When coding to the tumour, E34.0 may be used as an optional additional code to identify the functional activity.

E64.- Sequelae of malnutrition and other nutritional deficiencies

E68 Sequelae of hyperalimentation

These codes are not to be used as the preferred code for the "main condition" if the nature of the residual condition is recorded. When coding to the residual condition, E64.- or E68 may be used as an optional additional code.

Chapter V: Mental and behavioural disorders

The definitions of the categories and subcategories in this chapter are provided to assist the health care practitioner in establishing diagnostic labels; they should not be used by coders. The "main condition" code should be assigned on the basis of the diagnosis recorded by the practitioner, even if there appears to be a conflict between the condition as recorded and the definition. In some categories there is provision for optional additional codes.

Chapter VI: Diseases of the nervous system

Certain conditions classifiable to this chapter may result from the effects of drugs or other external causes. Codes from Chapter XX may be used as optional additional codes.

G09 Sequelae of inflammatory diseases of central nervous system

This code is not to be used as the preferred code for the "main condition" if the nature of the residual condition is recorded. When coding to the residual condition, G09 may be used as an optional additional code. Note that sequelae of categories G01[*], G02[*], G05[*] and G07[*] should not be assigned to G09, but rather to the categories established for sequelae of the underlying condition, e.g. B90-B94. If there is no sequelae category for the underlying condition, code to the underlying condition itself.

Example 14:   Main condition: Deafness due to tuberculous
                                   meningitis
                Specialty: Speech and hearing clinic

Code hearing loss, unspecified (H91.9) as the "main condition". B90.0 (Sequelae of central nervous system tuberculosis) may be used as an optional additional code.

Example 15:   Main condition: Epilepsy due to old brain abscess
                Specialty: Neurology

Code epilepsy, unspecified (G40.9) as the "main condition". G09 (Sequelae of inflammatory diseases of central nervous system) may be used as an optional additional code.

Example 16:   Main condition: Mild mental retardation after
                                   postimmunization encephalitis
                Specialty: Psychiatry

Code mild mental retardation (F70.9) as the "main condition". G09 (Sequelae of inflammatory diseases of central nervous system) may be used as an optional additional code.

G81-G83 *Paralytic syndromes*

These codes are not to be used as the preferred code for the "main condition" if a current cause is recorded, unless the episode of care was mainly for the paralysis itself. When coding to the cause, G81-G83 may be used as optional additional codes.

Example 17:   Main condition: Cerebrovascular accident with
                                   hemiplegia
                Other conditions: —
                Specialty: Neurology

Code stroke, not specified as haemorrhage or infarction (I64) as "main condition". G81.9 (Hemiplegia, unspecified) may be used as an optional additional code.

Example 18:   Main condition: Cerebral infarction three years ago
                Other conditions: Paralysis of left leg
                Patient receiving physical therapy

Code monoplegia of lower limb (G83.1) as "main condition". I69.3 (Sequelae of cerebral infarction) may be used as an optional additional code.

Chapter VII: Diseases of the eye and adnexa

H54.- Blindness and low vision

This code is not to be used as the preferred code for the "main condition" if the cause is recorded, unless the episode of care was mainly for the blindness itself. When coding to the cause, H54.- may be used as an optional additional code.

Chapter VIII: Diseases of the ear and mastoid process

H90-H91 Hearing loss

These codes are not to be used as the preferred code for the "main condition" if the cause is recorded, unless the episode of care was mainly for the hearing loss itself. When coding to the cause, H90.- or H91.- may be used as an optional additional code.

Chapter IX: Diseases of the circulatory system

I15.- Secondary hypertension

This code is not to be used as the preferred code for the "main condition" if the cause is recorded, unless the episode of care was mainly for the hypertension. When coding to the cause, I15.- may be used as an optional additional code.

I69.- Sequelae of cerebrovascular disease

This code is not to be used as the preferred code for the "main condition" if the nature of the residual condition is recorded. When coding to the residual condition, I69.- may be used as an optional additional code.

Chapter XV: Pregnancy, childbirth and the puerperium

O08.- Complications following abortion and ectopic and molar pregnancy

This code is not to be used as the preferred code for the "main condition", except where a new episode of care is solely for treatment of a complication, e.g. a current complication of a previous abortion. It may be used as an optional additional code with categories O00-O02 to identify associated complications and with categories O03-O07 to give fuller details of the complication.

Note that the inclusion terms provided at the subcategories of O08 should be referred to when assigning the fourth-character subcategories of O03-O07.

Example 19:   Main condition: Ruptured tubal pregnancy with shock
                 Specialty: Gynaecology

Code ruptured tubal pregnancy (O00.1) as the "main condition". O08.3 (Shock following abortion and ectopic and molar pregnancy) may be used as an optional additional code.

Example 20:   Main condition: Incomplete abortion with perforation
                                      of uterus
                 Specialty: Gynaecology

Code incomplete abortion with other and unspecified complications (O06.3) as the "main condition". Code O08.6 (Damage to pelvic organs and tissues following abortion and ectopic and molar pregnancy) may be added as an optional additional code.

Example 21:   Main condition: Disseminated intravascular
                                      coagulation following abortion
                                      performed two days ago at another
                                      facility
                 Specialty: Gynaecology

Code delayed or excessive haemorrhage following abortion and ectopic and molar pregnancy (O08.1). No other code is required since the abortion was performed during a previous episode of care.

O80-O84 Delivery

Use of these codes to describe the "main condition" should be limited to cases where the only information recorded is a statement of delivery or the method of delivery. Codes O80-O84 may be used as optional additional codes to indicate a method or type of delivery where no separate data item or procedural classification is being used for this purpose.

Example 22:   Main condition: Pregnancy
                 Other conditions: —
                 Procedure: Low forceps delivery

Code low forceps delivery (O81.0) as "main condition" since no other information is provided.

Example 23: Main condition: Pregnancy delivered
           Other conditions: Failed trial of labour
           Procedure: Caesarean section

Code failed trial of labour, unspecified (O66.4) as the "main condition". The code for caesarean section delivery, unspecified (O82.9), may be used as an optional additional code.

Example 24: Main condition: Twin pregnancy delivered
           Other conditions: —
           Procedure: Spontaneous delivery

Code twin pregnancy (O30.0) as the "main condition". O84.0 (Multiple delivery, all spontaneous) may be added as an optional additional code.

Example 25: Main condition: Term pregnancy delivered of dead fetus, 2800 g
           Other conditions: —
           Procedure: Spontaneous delivery

Code to maternal care for intrauterine death (O36.4) if no specific reason for the fetal death can be determined.

O98-O99 Maternal diseases classifiable elsewhere but complicating pregnancy, childbirth and the puerperium

The subcategories provided should be used as "main condition" codes in preference to categories outside Chapter XV when the conditions being classified have been indicated by the health care practitioner to have complicated the pregnant state, to have been aggravated by the pregnancy, or to have been the reason for obstetric care. The pertinent codes from other chapters may be used as optional additional codes to allow specification of the condition.

Example 26: Main condition: Toxoplasmosis
           Other conditions: Pregnancy undelivered
           Specialty: High-risk antenatal clinic

Code protozoal diseases complicating pregnancy, childbirth and the puerperium (O98.6) as the main condition. B58.9 (Toxoplasmosis, unspecified) may be used as an optional additional code to identify the specific organism.

Chapter XVIII: Symptoms, signs and abnormal clinical and laboratory findings, not elsewhere classified

Categories from this chapter should not be used as "main condition" codes unless the symptom, sign or abnormal finding was clearly the main condition treated or investigated during an episode of care and was unrelated to other conditions recorded by the health care practitioner. See also Rule MB3 (4.4.3) and the introduction to Chapter XVIII in Volume 1 for further information.

Chapter XIX: Injury, poisoning and certain other consequences of external causes

Where multiple injuries are recorded and no one of these has been selected as the "main condition", code to one of the categories provided for statements of multiple injuries of:

- same type to the same body region (usually fourth character .7 in categories S00-S99);
- different types to the same body region (usually fourth character .7 in the last category of each block, i.e. S09, S19, S29, etc.); and
- same type to different body regions (T00-T05).

Note the following exceptions:

- for internal injuries recorded with superficial injuries and/or open wounds only, code to internal injuries as the "main condition";
- for fractures of skull and facial bones with associated intracranial injury, code to the intracranial injury as the "main condition";
- for intracranial haemorrhage recorded with other injuries to the head only, code to intracranial haemorrhage as the "main condition"; and
- for fractures recorded with open wounds of the same location only, code to fracture as the "main condition".

When the multiple injury categories are used, codes for any individual injuries listed may be used as optional additional codes. In the case of the exceptions mentioned, in addition to the main condition code, the associated injury may be identified either by an optional additional code or by one of the digits provided for this purpose.

Example 27:	Main condition:	Injury of bladder and urethra
	Other conditions:	—

Code to injury of multiple pelvic organs (S37.7) as the "main condition". S37.2 (Injury of bladder) and S37.3 (Injury of urethra) may be used as optional additional codes.

Example 28:   Main condition: Open intracranial wound with
                                     cerebellar haemorrhage
                Other conditions: —

Code to traumatic cerebellar haemorrhage (S06.8) as the
"main condition". The open intracranial wound may be
indicated, if desired, by the addition of the code S01.9 (Open
wound of head, part unspecified) or by the addition of the
digit 1 (with open intracranial wound) to code S06.8
(S06.8.1).

T90-T98 Sequelae of injuries, of poisoning and of other consequences of external causes

These codes are not to be used as the preferred codes for "main condition" if
the nature of the residual conditions is recorded. When coding to the residual
condition, T90-T98 may be used as optional additional codes.

Chapter XX: External causes of morbidity and mortality

These codes are not to be used as "main condition" codes. They are intended
for use as optional additional codes to identify the external cause of
conditions classified in Chapter XIX, and may also be used as optional
additional codes with conditions classified in any other chapter but having an
external cause.

5. Statistical presentation

5.1 Introduction

This section presents the regulations regarding statistics for international comparison, and guidelines on data presentation in national and subnational statistical tables.

Those responsible for the analysis of the data should be involved in the development of the protocol for processing (including coding), not only of the diagnostic data but also of the other items to be cross-tabulated with them.

5.2 Source of data

The medical certification of the cause of death is normally the responsibility of the attending physician. The medical certificate of cause of death should be in line with the international recommendation (see section 4.1.3). Administrative procedures should ensure the confidentiality of data from the death certificate or other medical records.

In the case of deaths certified by coroners or other legal authorities, the medical evidence supplied to the certifier should be stated on the certificate in addition to any legal findings.

5.3 Level of detail of cause in tabulations

There are standard ways of listing causes coded according to the ICD, and there are formal recommendations concerning lists for tabulation permitting international comparison (see section 5.6). In other tabulations, the hierarchical structure of the ICD allows considerable flexibility for possible groupings.

The three- and four-character rubrics of the ICD allow for considerable detail. They are sometimes used to produce reference tables covering a whole range of data, which may not be published but retained in a central office where, on request, information can be extracted concerning specific diagnoses. The classification at this level is also used by specialists interested in the detailed study of a limited range of diagnoses. For these, more detail may be added at the fifth or even sixth character level, where coding has been done either to the supplementary characters given for some rubrics of the ICD or to one of the specialty-based adaptations of the family of classifications.

Although every effort has been made to ensure that the titles of ICD four-character subcategories are meaningful when they stand alone, they occasionally need to be read in conjunction with the three-character category title. Where this is so, it is necessary either to include the three-character rubrics (and their totals) or to use specially adapted titles for the four-character rubrics, which are intelligible when they stand alone. There are over 2000 rubrics at the three-character level, identifying all conditions likely to be of public health interest.

There are also special tabulation lists in Volume 1 which are intended for circumstances in which the three-character list is too detailed, and are designed so that international comparison of significant diseases and groups of diseases is not frustrated by different groupings having been used in different countries.

5.4   The recommended special tabulation lists for mortality

The special tabulation lists for mortality are given in Volume 1.

5.4.1   The condensed lists

The two condensed lists, List 1 and List 3, provide items for each ICD chapter and also, within most chapters, identify the items of the selected lists together with residual items entitled "Remainder of...", which complete the coverage of the respective chapter. They thus condense the full range of ICD three-character categories into a manageable number of items for many publication purposes.

5.4.2   The selected lists

The two selected lists, List 2 and List 4, contain items within most ICD chapters, for conditions and external causes significant for the monitoring and analysis of population health status and mortality-related health concerns at both national and international levels. Chapter totals are not provided and only a few chapters have residual rubrics that enable such totals to be obtained.

5.4.3   Use of prefixes to identify the mortality lists

Use of the numerical prefixes to the item numbers prevents confusion between the special tabulation lists where items for the same condition carry different numbers. (The item numbers can be distinguished from ICD four-character codes which have a letter in the first position.) Where an adapted list is used for national or subnational purposes, an alternative identifying prefix should be used.

5.4.4   Locally designed lists

The four special tabulation lists provide for most countries an adequate source of information about the most important diseases and external causes of death. They also facilitate comparison over time and observation of shifts in the relative frequencies of, for example, infectious diseases and degenerative diseases, as health programmes take effect. They permit comparison between subnational areas and population subgroups. In addition, they make possible meaningful international comparisons of causes of death.

When there is no need for international comparison, lists similar to the special tabulation lists can be designed for use locally. The ICD rubrics of such lists can be selected and grouped in whatever way is most appropriate and useful. Special lists would be needed, for example, for monitoring the progress, in terms of morbidity and mortality, of many local health programmes.

When adapting the special tabulation lists to national requirements, or when a tabulation list is being devised for a new or special project, it is helpful to have a test run, simply counting the number of cases falling into each three-character category, to determine for which conditions grouping to broad rubrics is appropriate and where the use of subcategories could be necessary.

Where a local list is constructed, the key to the condensed categories should contain the three (or four) character codes of the core classification.

5.5   The special tabulation list for morbidity

5.5.1   Description

The tabulation list for morbidity contains 298 detailed items. The morbidity list is a condensed list in which each category is included only once and totals for groups of diseases and ICD chapters can be obtained by the addition of sequential items.

The morbidity list is intended as a basis for national lists and for intercountry comparison. National lists can be constructed by either condensing or expanding the core classification as appropriate. The list is suitable for data on inpatient care and, with suitable adaptation - notably aggregation of some items and expansion of items relating to Chapter XVIII (Symptoms, signs and abnormal clinical and laboratory findings) and Chapter XXI (Factors influencing health status and contact with health services) - for information from other sources, such as ambulatory care and surveys. When a local list is constructed, the key to the condensed categories should contain the three (or four) character codes of the core classification.

The morbidity list includes the code numbers of asterisk categories for use when the asterisk code for dual classification is included in the analysis. The list can be used for either dagger-based or asterisk-based tabulations and it is important, therefore, to indicate in each table which basis has been used.

5.5.2 Modification of the special tabulation list for morbidity according to national requirements

If, after examination of the frequencies of the ICD three-character rubrics, it is felt necessary to expand the list, some of the items for a range of ICD categories can be subdivided according to the core classification or even to the four-character level. If the recommended list is considered to be too detailed or if a shorter list is required, selection can be made based on national or local health concerns. Depending on a country's "epidemiological profile", categories may be combined to shorten the list.

5.6 Recommendations in relation to statistical tables for international comparison

5.6.1 Statistical tables

The degree of detail in cross-classification by cause, sex, age, and geographical area will depend both on the purpose and range of the statistics and on the practical limits to their tabulation. The following patterns, which are designed to promote international compatibility, present standard ways of expressing various characteristics. Where a different classification is used in published tables (e.g. in age-grouping), it should be reducible to one of the recommended groupings.

(a) Analysis by the International Classification of Diseases should, as appropriate, be in accordance with:
  (i)   the detailed list of three-character categories, with or without four-character subcategories;
  (ii) one of the special tabulation lists for mortality;
  (iii) the special tabulation list for morbidity.
(b) Age classification for general purposes:
  (i)   under 1 year, single years to 4 years, 5-year groups from 5 to 84 years, 85 years and over;
  (ii) under 1 year, 1-4 years, 5-14 years, 15-24 years, 25-34 years, 35-44 years, 45-54 years, 55-64 years, 65-74 years, 75 years and over.
  (iii) under 1 year, 1-14 years, 15-44 years, 45-64 years, 65 years and over.
(c) Classification by area should, as appropriate, be in accordance with:
  (i)   each major civil division;
  (ii) each town or conurbation of 1 000 000 population and over, otherwise the largest town with a population of at least 100 000;
  (iii) a national aggregate of urban areas of 100 000 population and over;
  (iv) a national aggregate of urban areas of less than 100 000 population;
  (v)   a national aggregate of rural areas.

Note 1. Statistics relating to (c) should include the definitions of urban and rural used.

Note 2. In countries where medical certification of the cause of death is incomplete or limited to certain areas, figures for deaths not medically certified should be published separately.

5.6.2 Tabulation of causes of death

Statistics of causes of death for a defined area should be in accordance with recommendation (a)(i) above, or, if this is not possible, with recommendation (a)(ii). Deaths should preferably be classified by sex and age group as in recommendation (b)(i).

Statistics of causes of deaths for the areas in recommendation (c) should comply with recommendation (a)(ii), or if this is not possible, with recommendation (a)(iii). They should preferably be tabulated by sex and age group as in recommendation (b)(ii).

5.7 Standards and reporting requirements related to fetal, perinatal, neonatal and infant mortality

The following definitions have been adopted by the World Health Assembly in relation both to statistics amenable to international comparison and to reporting requirements for the data from which they are derived. The definitions adopted by the Health Assembly appear in Volume 1 and, for convenience, are restated below.

5.7.1 Definitions

Live birth
Live birth is the complete expulsion or extraction from its mother of a product of conception, irrespective of the duration of the pregnancy, which, after such separation, breathes or shows any other evidence of life, such as beating of the heart, pulsation of the umbilical cord, or definite movement of voluntary muscles, whether or not the umbilical cord has been cut or the placenta is attached; each product of such a birth is considered liveborn.

Fetal death [deadborn fetus]
Fetal death is death prior to the complete expulsion or extraction from its mother of a product of conception, irrespective of the duration of pregnancy; the death is indicated by the fact that after such separation the fetus does not breathe or show any other evidence of life, such as beating of the heart, pulsation of the umbilical cord, or definite movement of voluntary muscles.

Birth weight
The first weight of the fetus or newborn obtained after birth.

For live births, birth weight should preferably be measured within the first hour of life before significant postnatal weight loss has occurred. While statistical tabulations include 500 g groupings for birth weight, weights should not be recorded in those groupings. The actual weight should be recorded to the degree of accuracy to which it is measured.

The definitions of "low", "very low", and "extremely low" birth weight do not constitute mutually exclusive categories. Below the set limits they are all-inclusive and therefore overlap (i.e. "low" includes "very low" and "extremely low", while "very low" includes "extremely low").

Low birth weight
Less than 2500 g (up to and including 2499 g).

Very low birth weight
Less than 1500 g (up to and including 1499 g).

Extremely low birth weight
Less than 1000 g (up to and including 999 g).

Gestational age
The duration of gestation is measured from the first day of the last normal menstrual period. Gestational age is expressed in completed days or completed weeks (e.g. events occurring 280 to 286 completed days after the onset of the last normal menstrual period are considered to have occurred at 40 weeks of gestation).

Gestational age is frequently a source of confusion, when calculations are based on menstrual dates. For the purposes of calculation of gestational age from the date of the first day of the last normal menstrual period and the date of delivery, it should be borne in mind that the first day is day zero and not day one; days 0-6 therefore correspond to "completed week zero"; days 7-13 to "completed week one"; and the 40th week of actual gestation is synonymous with "completed week 39". Where the date of the last normal menstrual period is not available, gestational age should be based on the best clinical estimate. In order to avoid misunderstanding, tabulations should indicate both weeks and days.

Pre-term
Less than 37 completed weeks (less than 259 days) of gestation.

Term
From 37 completed weeks to less than 42 completed weeks (259 to 293 days) of gestation.

Post-term
42 completed weeks or more (294 days or more) of gestation.

Perinatal period
The perinatal period commences at 22 completed weeks (154 days) of gestation (the time when birth weight is normally 500 g), and ends seven completed days after birth.

Neonatal period
The neonatal period commences at birth and ends 28 completed days after birth. Neonatal deaths (deaths among live births during the first 28 completed days of life) may be subdivided into early neonatal deaths, occurring during the first seven days of life, and late neonatal deaths, occurring after the seventh day but before 28 completed days of life.

Age at death during the first day of life (day zero) should be recorded in units of completed minutes or hours of life. For the second (day 1), third (day 2) and through 27 completed days of life, age at death should be recorded in days.

5.7.2 Reporting criteria

The legal requirements for the registration of fetal deaths and live births vary from country to country and even within countries. If possible, all fetuses and infants weighing at least 500 g at birth, whether alive or dead, should be included in the statistics. When information on birth weight is unavailable, the corresponding criteria for gestational age (22 completed weeks) or body length (25 cm crown-heel) should be used. The criteria for deciding whether an event has taken place within the perinatal period should be applied in the order: (1) birth weight, (2) gestational age, (3) crown-heel length. The inclusion of fetuses and infants weighing between 500 g and 1000 g in national statistics is recommended both because of its inherent value and because it improves the coverage of reporting at 1000 g and over.

5.7.3 Statistics for international comparison

In statistics for international comparison, inclusion of the extremely low-birth-weight group disrupts the validity of comparisons and is not recommended. Countries should arrange registration and reporting procedures so that the events and the criteria for their inclusion in the statistics can be easily identified. Less mature fetuses and infants not corresponding to these criteria (i.e. weighing less than 1000 g) should be excluded from perinatal statistics unless there are legal or other valid reasons to the contrary, in which case their inclusion must be explicitly stated. Where birth weight, gestational age and crown-heel length are not known, the event should be included in, rather than excluded from, mortality statistics of the perinatal period. Countries should also present statistics in which both the numerator and the denominator of all ratios and rates are restricted to fetuses and infants weighing 1000 g or more (weight-specific ratios and rates); where information on birth weight is not available, the corresponding gestational age (28 completed weeks) or body length (35 cm crown-heel) should be used.

In reporting fetal, perinatal, neonatal and infant mortality statistics the number of deaths due to malformations should whenever possible be identified for live births and fetal deaths and in relation to birth weights of 500-999 g and 1000 g or more. Neonatal deaths due to malformations should be subdivided into early and late neonatal deaths. This information enables perinatal and neonatal mortality statistics to be reported with or without the deaths from malformations.

Ratios and rates

Published ratios and rates should always specify the denominator, i.e. live births or total births (live births plus fetal deaths). Countries are encouraged to provide the ratios and rates listed below, or as many of them as their data collection systems permit.

Fetal death ratio

$$\frac{\text{Fetal deaths}}{\text{Live births}} \times 1000$$

Fetal death rate

$$\frac{\text{Fetal deaths}}{\text{Total births}} \times 1000$$

Fetal death rate, weight-specific

$$\frac{\text{Fetal deaths weighing 1000 g and over}}{\text{Total births weighing 1000 g and over}} \times 1000$$

Early neonatal mortality rate

$$\frac{\text{Early neonatal deaths}}{\text{Live births}} \times 1000$$

Early neonatal mortality rate, weight-specific

$$\frac{\text{Early neonatal deaths of infants weighing 1000 g and over at birth}}{\text{Live births weighing 1000 g and over}} \times 1000$$

Perinatal mortality ratio

$$\frac{\text{Fetal deaths and early neonatal deaths}}{\text{Live births}} \times 1000$$

Perinatal mortality rate

$$\frac{\text{Fetal deaths and early neonatal deaths}}{\text{Total births}} \times 1000$$

The perinatal mortality rate is the number of deaths of fetuses weighing at least 500 g (or, when birth weight is unavailable, after 22 completed weeks of gestation or with a crown-heel length of 25 cm or more), plus the number of early neonatal deaths, per 1000 total births. Because of the different denominators in each component, this is not necessarily equal to the sum of the fetal death rate and the early neonatal mortality rate.

Perinatal mortality rate, weight-specific

$$\frac{\text{Fetal deaths weighing 1000 g and over, plus}}{\text{early neonatal deaths of infants weighing 1000 g and over at birth}}{\text{Total births weighing 1000 g and over}} \times 1000$$

Neonatal mortality rate

$$\frac{\text{Neonatal deaths}}{\text{Live births}} \times 1000$$

Neonatal mortality rate, weight-specific

$$\frac{\text{Neonatal deaths of infants weighing 1000 g and over at birth}}{\text{Live births weighing 1000 g and over}} \times 1000$$

Infant mortality rate

$$\frac{\text{Deaths under one year of age}}{\text{Live births}} \times 1000$$

Infant mortality rate, weight-specific

$$\frac{\text{Infant deaths among live births weighing 1000 g and over at birth}}{\text{Live births weighing 1000 g and over}} \times 1000$$

5.7.4 Presentation of causes of perinatal mortality

For statistics of perinatal mortality derived from the form of certificate recommended for this purpose (see section 4.3.1), full-scale multiple-cause analysis of all conditions reported will be of greatest benefit. Where such analysis is impracticable, analysis of the main disease or condition in the fetus or infant (part (a)) and of the main maternal condition affecting the fetus or infant (part (c)) with cross-tabulation of groups of these two conditions should be regarded as the minimum. Where it is necessary to select only one condition (for example, when early neonatal deaths must be incorporated into single-cause tables of deaths at all ages), the main disease or condition in the fetus or infant (part (a)) should be selected.

Age classification for special statistics of infant mortality

(i) By single days for the first week of life (under 24 hours, 1, 2, 3, 4, 5, 6 days), 7-13 days, 14-20 days, 21-27 days, 28 days and up to, but not including, 2 months, by single months of life from 2 months to 1 year (2, 3, 4 ... 11 months).

(ii) Under 24 hours, 1-6 days, 7-27 days, 28 days up to, but not including, 3 months, 3-5 months, 6 months but under 1 year.

(iii) Under 7 days, 7-27 days, 28 days but under 1 year.

Age classification for early neonatal deaths

(i) Under 1 hour, 1-11 hours, 12-23 hours, 24-47 hours, 48-71 hours, 72-167 hours;

(ii) Under 1 hour, 1-23 hours, 24-167 hours.

Birth weight classification for perinatal mortality statistics

By weight intervals of 500 g, i.e. 1000-1499 g, etc.

Gestational age classification for perinatal mortality statistics

Under 28 weeks (under 196 days), 28-31 weeks (196-223 days), 32-36 weeks (224-258 days), 37-41 weeks (259-293 days), 42 weeks and over (294 days and over).

5.8 Standards and reporting requirements related to maternal mortality

5.8.1 Definitions

Maternal death

A maternal death is the death of a woman while pregnant or within 42 days of termination of pregnancy, irrespective of the duration and the site of the pregnancy, from any cause related to or aggravated by the pregnancy or its management, but not from accidental or incidental causes.

Late maternal death

A late maternal death is the death of a woman from direct or indirect obstetric causes more than 42 days but less than one year after termination of pregnancy.

Pregnancy-related death

A pregnancy-related death is the death of a woman while pregnant or within 42 days of termination of pregnancy, irrespective of the cause of death.

Maternal deaths should be subdivided into two groups:

Direct obstetric deaths: those resulting from obstetric complications of the pregnant state (pregnancy, labour and puerperium), from interventions, omissions, incorrect treatment, or from a chain of events resulting from any of the above.

Indirect obstetric deaths: those resulting from previous existing disease or disease that developed during pregnancy and which was not due to direct obstetric causes, but which was aggravated by physiologic effects of pregnancy.

In order to improve the quality of maternal mortality data and provide alternative methods of collecting data on deaths during pregnancy or related to it, as well as to encourage the recording of deaths from obstetric causes occurring more than 42 days following termination of pregnancy, the Forty-third World Health Assembly in 1990 adopted the recommendation that countries consider the inclusion on death certificates of questions regarding current pregnancy and pregnancy within one year preceding death.

5.8.2   International reporting

For the purpose of the international reporting of maternal mortality, only those maternal deaths occurring before the end of the 42-day reference period should be included in the calculation of the various ratios and rates, although the recording of later deaths is useful for national analytical purposes.

5.8.3   Published maternal mortality rates

Published maternal mortality rates should always specify the numerator (number of recorded maternal deaths), which can be given as:

- the number of recorded direct obstetric deaths, or
- the number of recorded obstetric deaths (direct plus indirect).

It should be noted that maternal deaths from HIV disease (B20-B24) and obstetrical tetanus (A34) are coded to Chapter I. Care must be taken to include such cases in the maternal mortality rate.

5.8.4   Denominators for maternal mortality

The denominator used for calculating maternal mortality should be specified as either the number of live births or the number of total births (live births plus fetal deaths). Where both denominators are available, a calculation should be published for each.

Ratios and rates

Results should be expressed as a ratio of the numerator to the denominator, multiplied by k (where k may be 1000, 10 000 or 100 000, as preferred and indicated by the country). Maternal mortality ratios and rates can thus be expressed as follows:

Maternal mortality rate[1]

$$\frac{\text{Maternal deaths (direct and indirect)}}{\text{Live births}} \times k$$

Direct obstetric mortality ratio

$$\frac{\text{Direct obstetric deaths only}}{\text{Live births}} \times k$$

Pregnancy-related mortality ratio

$$\frac{\text{Pregnancy-related deaths}}{\text{Live births}} \times k$$

5.9 Proportion of deaths classified to ill-defined causes

The allocation of a high proportion of causes of death to Chapter XVIII (Symptoms, signs, and abnormal clinical and laboratory findings, not elsewhere classified) indicates a need to check or estimate the quality of the tabulated data allocated to more specific causes assigned to other chapters.

5.10 Morbidity

There are a wide variety of possible sources of information on morbidity. The data most suitable for analysis on a national or regional basis are those that enable some calculation to be made of the incidence of diseases, or at least of those diseases coming, for example, under medical or hospital care. It is primarily for data on episodes of health care that the formally agreed

---

[1] The use of the term "rate", although inexact in this context, is retained for the sake of continuity.

guidelines and definitions for recording causes of morbidity and selection of a single condition, where appropriate, are intended. Other types of data require the development of local rules.

The problems of morbidity statistics start with the very definition of "morbidity". There is much scope for improving morbidity statistics. International comparisons of morbidity data are, at present, feasible only to a very limited extent and for clearly defined purposes. National or regional information on morbidity has to be interpreted in relation to its source and with background knowledge of the quality of the data, diagnostic reliability, and demographic and socioeconomic characteristics.

5.11 Precautions needed when tabulation lists include subtotals

It may not always be apparent to those processing the data that some of the items in the tabulation lists are in fact subtotals; for instance, titles of blocks and, in the case of the four-character list of ICD-10, titles of three-character categories, as well as the items for chapter titles in the condensed versions of the mortality tabulation lists. These entries should be ignored when totals are calculated, otherwise cases would be counted more than once.

5.12 Problems of a small population

Population size is one of the factors that has to be considered when the health status of a population is assessed by means of mortality or morbidity data. In countries with small populations, the annual numbers of events in many categories of the short lists will be very small, and will fluctuate randomly from year to year. This is especially so for separate age groups and sexes. The problems can be alleviated by one or more of the following measures:

- use or presentation of broad groupings of ICD rubrics, such as chapters;
- aggregation of data over a longer period, e.g. to take the preceding two years' data together with those for the current year and produce a "moving average" figure;
- using the broadest of the age groupings recommended at 5.6.1 and 5.7.4.

What applies for small national populations also holds true in general for subnational segments of larger populations. Investigations of health issues in population subgroups have to take into consideration the effect of the size of each of the subgroups on the type of analysis used. This need is generally recognized when dealing with sample surveys, but often overlooked when the investigation concerns the health problems of special groups in the national population.

5.13 "Empty cells" and cells with low frequencies

Whatever list of causes is being used, it may be found that no cases occur in certain cells of a statistical table. Where there are many empty lines in a table, it is worth considering the omission of such lines from a published table or from a computer printout. When only the occasional case of a disease occurs in a country, the line can be regularly omitted from the published table and a footnote added to indicate either that there were no cases or, when sporadic cases do occur, in which cell the case would have appeared.

For cells with very low frequencies, especially those relating to diseases that would not be expected to occur, it is important to establish that the cases existed and did not result from a coding or processing error. This should be carried out as part of the general quality control of the data.

6. History of the development of the ICD[1]

6.1 Early history

Sir George Knibbs, the eminent Australian statistician, credited François Bossier de Lacroix (1706-1777), better known as Sauvages, with the first attempt to classify diseases systematically (*10*). Sauvages' comprehensive treatise was published under the title *Nosologia methodica*. A contemporary of Sauvages was the great methodologist Linnaeus (1707-1778), one of whose treatises was entitled *Genera morborum*. At the beginning of the 19th century, the classification of disease in most general use was one by William Cullen (1710-1790), of Edinburgh, which was published in 1785 under the title *Synopsis nosologiae methodicae*.

For all practical purposes, however, the statistical study of disease began a century earlier with the work of John Graunt on the London Bills of Mortality. The kind of classification envisaged by this pioneer is exemplified by his attempt to estimate the proportion of liveborn children who died before reaching the age of six years, no records of age at death being available. He took all deaths classed as thrush, convulsions, rickets, teeth and worms, abortives, chrysomes, infants, livergrown, and overlaid and added to them half the deaths classed as smallpox, swinepox, measles, and worms without convulsions.Despite the crudity of this classification his estimate of a 36% mortality before the age of six years appears from later evidence to have been a good one. While three centuries have contributed something to the scientific accuracy of disease classification, there are many who doubt the usefulness of attempts to compile statistics of disease, or even causes of death, because of the difficulties of classification. To these, one can quote Major Greenwood: "The scientific purist, who will wait for medical statistics until they are nosologically exact, is no wiser than Horace's rustic waiting for the river to flow away" (*11*).

Fortunately for the progress of preventive medicine, the General Register Office of England and Wales, at its inception in 1837, found in William Farr (1807-1883) - its first medical statistician - a man who not only made the best

---

[1] Most of the material presented in sections 6.1-6.3 is reproduced from the Introduction to the Seventh Revision of the ICD, which gives an excellent description of the early history of the classification.

possible use of the imperfect classifications of disease available at the time, but laboured to secure better classifications and international uniformity in their use.

Farr found the classification of Cullen in use in the public services of his day. It had not been revised to embody the advances of medical science, nor was it deemed by him to be satisfactory for statistical purposes. In the first Annual Report of the Registrar General (12), therefore, he discussed the principles that should govern a statistical classification of disease and urged the adoption of a uniform classification as follows:

> The advantages of a uniform statistical nomenclature, however imperfect, are so obvious, that it is surprising no attention has been paid to its enforcement in Bills of Mortality. Each disease has, in many instances, been denoted by three or four terms, and each term has been applied to as many different diseases: vague, inconvenient names have been employed, or complications have been registered instead of primary diseases. The nomenclature is of as much importance in this department of inquiry as weights and measures in the physical sciences, and should be settled without delay.

Both nomenclature and statistical classification received constant study and consideration by Farr in his annual "Letters" to the Registrar General published in the Annual Reports of the Registrar General. The utility of a uniform classification of causes of death was so strongly recognized at the first International Statistical Congress, held in Brussels in 1853, that the Congress requested William Farr and Marc d'Espine, of Geneva, to prepare an internationally applicable, uniform classification of causes of death. At the next Congress, in Paris in 1855, Farr and d'Espine submitted two separate lists which were based on very different principles. Farr's classification was arranged under five groups: epidemic diseases, constitutional (general) diseases, local diseases arranged according to anatomical site, developmental diseases, and diseases that are the direct result of violence. D'Espine classified diseases according to their nature (gouty, herpetic, haematic, etc.). The Congress adopted a compromise list of 139 rubrics. In 1864, this classification was revised in Paris on the basis of Farr's model and was subsequently further revised in 1874, 1880, and 1886. Although this classification was never universally accepted, the general arrangement proposed by Farr, including the principle of classifying diseases by anatomical site, survived as the basis of the International List of Causes of Death.

6.2   Adoption of the International List of Causes of Death

The International Statistical Institute, the successor to the International Statistical Congress, at its meeting in Vienna in 1891, charged a committee, chaired by Jacques Bertillon (1851-1922), Chief of Statistical Services of the City of Paris, with the preparation of a classification of causes of death. It is of interest to note that Bertillon was the grandson of Achille Guillard, a noted botanist and statistician, who had introduced the resolution requesting Farr and d'Espine to prepare a uniform classification at the first International Statistical Congress in 1853. The report of this committee was presented by Bertillon at the meeting of the International Statistical Institute in Chicago in 1893 and adopted by it. The classification prepared by Bertillon's committee was based on the classification of causes of death used by the City of Paris, which, since its revision in 1885, represented a synthesis of English, German, and Swiss classifications. The classification was based on the principle, adopted by Farr, of distinguishing between general diseases and those localized to a particular organ or anatomical site. In accordance with the instructions of the Vienna Congress made at the suggestion of L. Guillaume, the Director of the Federal Bureau of Statistics of Switzerland, Bertillon included three classifications: the first, an abridged classification of 44 titles; the second, a classification of 99 titles; and the third, a classification of 161 titles.

The Bertillon Classification of Causes of Death, as it was first called, received general approval and was adopted by several countries, as well as by many cities. The classification was first used in North America by Jesus E. Monjaras for the statistics of San Luis de Potosi, Mexico (*13*). In 1898, the American Public Health Association, at its meeting in Ottawa, Canada, recommended the adoption of the Bertillon Classification by registrars of Canada, Mexico, and the United States of America. The Association further suggested that the classification should be revised every ten years.

At the meeting of the International Statistical Institute at Christiania in 1899, Bertillon presented a report on the progress of the classification, including the recommendations of the American Public Health Association for decennial revisions. The International Statistical Institute then adopted the following resolution (*14*):

> The International Statistical Institute, convinced of the necessity of using in the different countries comparable nomenclatures:
>
> Learns with pleasure of the adoption by all the statistical offices of North America, by some of those of South America, and by some in Europe, of the system of cause of death nomenclature presented in 1893;

Insists vigorously that this system of nomenclature be adopted in principle and without revision, by all the statistical institutions of Europe;

Approves, at least in its general lines, the system of decennial revision proposed by the American Public Health Association at its Ottawa session (1898):

Urges the statistical offices who have not yet adhered, to do so without delay, and to contribute to the comparability of the cause of death nomenclature.

The French Government therefore convoked in Paris, in August 1900, the first International Conference for the Revision of the Bertillon or International List of Causes of Death. Delegates from 26 countries attended this Conference. A detailed classification of causes of death consisting of 179 groups and an abridged classification of 35 groups were adopted on 21 August 1900. The desirability of decennial revisions was recognized, and the French Government was requested to call the next meeting in 1910. In fact the next conference was held in 1909, and the Government of France called succeeding conferences in 1920, 1929, and 1938.

Bertillon continued to be the guiding force in the promotion of the International List of Causes of Death, and the revisions of 1900, 1910, and 1920 were carried out under his leadership. As Secretary-General of the International Conference, he sent out the provisional revision for 1920 to more than 500 people, asking for comments. His death in 1922 left the International Conference without a guiding hand.

At the 1923 session of the International Statistical Institute, Michel Huber, Bertillon's successor in France, recognized this lack of leadership and introduced a resolution for the International Statistical Institute to renew its stand of 1893 in regard to the International Classification of Causes of Death and to cooperate with other international organizations in preparation for subsequent revisions. The Health Organization of the League of Nations had also taken an active interest in vital statistics and appointed a Commission of Statistical Experts to study the classification of diseases and causes of death, as well as other problems in the field of medical statistics. E. Roesle, Chief of the Medical Statistical Service of the German Health Bureau and a member of the Commission of Expert Statisticians, prepared a monograph that listed the expansion in the rubrics of the 1920 International List of Causes of Death that would be required if the classification was to be used in the tabulation of statistics of morbidity. This careful study was published by the Health Organization of the League of Nations in 1928 (15). In order to coordinate the work of both agencies, an international commission, known as the "Mixed Commission", was created with an equal number of representatives from the International Statistical Institute and the Health Organization of the League of Nations. This Commission drafted the proposals for the Fourth

(1929) and the Fifth (1938) revisions of the International List of Causes of Death.

6.3   The Fifth Decennial Revision Conference

The Fifth International Conference for the Revision of the International List of Causes of Death, like the preceding conferences, was convened by the Government of France and was held in Paris in October 1938. The Conference approved three lists: a detailed list of 200 titles, an intermediate list of 87 titles and an abridged list of 44 titles. Apart from bringing the lists up to date in accordance with the progress of science, particularly in the chapter on infectious and parasitic diseases, and changes in the chapters on puerperal conditions and on accidents, the Conference made as few changes as possible in the contents, number, and even in the numbering of the items. A list of causes of stillbirth was also drawn up and approved by the Conference.

As regards classification of diseases for morbidity statistics, the Conference recognized the growing need for a corresponding list of diseases to meet the statistical requirements of widely differing organizations, such as health insurance organizations, hospitals, military medical services, health administrations, and similar bodies. The following resolution, therefore, was adopted (*16*):

2. International Lists of Diseases.

In view of the importance of the compilation of international lists of diseases corresponding to the international lists of causes of death:

The Conference recommends that the Joint Committee appointed by the International Institute of Statistics and the Health Organization of the League of Nations undertake, as in 1929, the preparation of international lists of diseases, in conjunction with experts and representatives of the organizations specially concerned.

Pending the compilation of international lists of diseases, the Conference recommends that the various national lists in use should, as far as possible, be brought into line with the detailed International List of Causes of Death (the numbers of the chapters, headings and subheadings in the said List being given in brackets).

The Conference further recommended that the United States Government continue its studies of the statistical treatment of joint causes of death in the following resolution (*16*):

3. Death Certificate and Selection of Causes of Death where more than One Cause is given (Joint Causes)

The Conference,

Whereas, in 1929, the United States Government was good enough to undertake the study of the means of unifying the methods of selection of the main cause of death to be tabulated in those cases where two or more causes are mentioned on the death certificate,

And whereas, the numerous surveys completed or in the course of preparation in several countries reveal the importance of this problem, which has not yet been solved,

And whereas, according to these surveys, the international comparability of death rates from the various diseases requires, not only the solution of the problem of the selection of the main tabulated cause of death, but also the solution of a number of other questions;

(1) Warmly thanks the United States Government for the work it has accomplished or promoted in this connection;

(2) Requests the United States Government to continue its investigations during the next ten years, in co-operation with other countries and organizations, on a slightly wider basis, and

(3) Suggests that, for these future investigations, the United States Government should set up a subcommittee comprising representatives of countries and organizations participating in the investigations undertaken in this connection.

6.4 Previous classifications of diseases for morbidity statistics

In the discussion so far, classification of disease has been presented almost wholly in relation to cause-of-death statistics. Farr, however, recognized that it was desirable "to extend the same system of nomenclature to diseases which, though not fatal, cause disability in the population, and now figure in the tables of the diseases of armies, navies, hospitals, prisons, lunatic asylums, public institutions of every kind, and sickness societies, as well as in the census of countries like Ireland, where the diseases of all the people are enumerated" (*9*). In his *Report on nomenclature and statistical classification of diseases*, presented to the Second International Statistical Congress, he therefore included in the general list of diseases most of those diseases that affect health as well as diseases that are fatal. At the Fourth International Statistical Congress, held in London in 1860, Florence Nightingale urged the adoption of Farr's classification of diseases for the tabulation of hospital morbidity in the paper, *Proposals for a uniform plan of hospital statistics.*

At the First International Conference to revise the Bertillon Classification of Causes of Death in Paris in 1900, a parallel classification of diseases for use in statistics of sickness was adopted. A parallel list was also adopted at the second conference in 1909. The extra categories for non-fatal diseases were formed by subdivision of certain rubrics of the cause-of-death classification into two or three disease groups, each of these being designated by a letter. The translation in English of the Second Decennial Revision, published by the United States Department of Commerce and Labor in 1910, was entitled *International Classification of Causes of Sickness and Death.* Later revisions incorporated some of the groups into the detailed International List of Causes of Death. The Fourth International Conference adopted a classification of illness which differed from the detailed International List of Causes of Death only by the addition of further subdivisions of 12 titles. These international classifications of illnesses, however, failed to receive general acceptance, as they provided only a limited expansion of the basic cause-of-death list.

In the absence of a uniform classification of diseases that could be used satisfactorily for statistics of illness, many countries found it necessary to prepare their own lists. A Standard Morbidity Code was prepared by the Dominion Council of Health of Canada and published in 1936. The main subdivisions of this code represented the eighteen chapters of the 1929 Revision of the International List of Causes of Death, and these were subdivided into some 380 specific disease categories. At the Fifth International Conference in 1938, the Canadian delegate introduced a modification of this list for consideration as the basis for an international list of causes of illness. Although no action was taken on this proposal, the Conference adopted the resolution quoted above.

In 1944, provisional classifications of diseases and injuries were published in both the United Kingdom and the United States of America for use in the tabulation of morbidity statistics. Both classifications were more extensive than the Canadian list, but, like it, followed the general order of diseases in the International List of Causes of Death. The British classification was prepared by the Committee on Hospital Morbidity Statistics of the Medical Research Council, which was created in January 1942. It is entitled *A provisional classification of diseases and injuries for use in compiling morbidity statistics (17).* It was prepared with the purpose of providing a scheme for collecting and recording statistics of patients admitted to hospitals in the United Kingdom, using a standard classification of diseases and injuries, and was used throughout the country by governmental and other agencies.

A few years earlier, in August 1940, the Surgeon-General of the United States Public Health Service and the Director of the United States Bureau of the Census published a list of diseases and injuries for tabulation of morbidity statistics (*18*). The code was prepared by the Division of Public Health Methods of the Public Health Service in cooperation with a committee of consultants appointed by the Surgeon-General. *The Manual for coding causes of illness according to a diagnosis code for tabulating morbidity statistics*, consisting of the diagnosis code, a tabular list of inclusions, and an alphabetical index, was published in 1944. The code was used in several hospitals, in a large number of voluntary hospital insurance plans and medical care plans, and in special studies by other agencies in the United States.

6.5   United States Committee on Joint Causes of Death

In compliance with the resolution of the Fifth International Conference, the American Secretary of State in 1945 appointed the United States Committee on Joint Causes of Death under the chairmanship of Lowell J. Reed, Professor of Biostatistics at Johns Hopkins University. Members and consultants of this committee included representatives of the Governments of Canada and the United Kingdom and the Health Section of the League of Nations. The committee recognized the general trend of thought with regard to lists of morbidity and mortality statistics, and decided that, before taking up the matter of joint causes, it would be advantageous to consider classifications from the point of view of morbidity and mortality, since the problem of joint causes pertained to both types of statistics.

The committee also took into account that part of the resolution on International Lists of Diseases of the previous International Conference recommending that the "various national lists in use should, as far as possible, be brought into line with the detailed International List of Causes of Death". It recognized that the classification of sickness and injury is closely linked with the classification of causes of death. The view that such lists are fundamentally different arises from the erroneous belief that the International List is a classification of terminal causes, whereas it is in fact based upon the morbid condition that initiated the train of events ultimately resulting in death. The committee believed that, in order to utilize fully both morbidity and mortality statistics, not only should the classification of diseases for both purposes be comparable, but if possible there should be a single list.

Furthermore, an increasing number of statistical organizations were using medical records involving both sickness and death. Even in organizations that compile only morbidity statistics, fatal as well as non-fatal cases must be coded. A single list, therefore, greatly facilitates their coding operations. It also provides a common base for comparison of morbidity and mortality statistics.

A subcommittee was therefore appointed, which prepared a draft of a Proposed Statistical Classification of Diseases, Injuries and Causes of Death. A final draft was adopted by the committee after it had been modified on the basis of trials undertaken by various agencies in Canada, the United Kingdom and the United States of America.

6.6 Sixth Revision of the International Lists

The International Health Conference held in New York City in June and July 1946 (*19*) entrusted the Interim Commission of the World Health Organization with the responsibility of:

> reviewing the existing machinery and of undertaking such preparatory work as may be necessary in connection with:
>
> (i) the next decennial revision of "The International Lists of Causes of Death" (including the lists adopted under the International Agreement of 1934, relating to Statistics of Causes of Death); and
>
> (ii) the establishment of International Lists of Causes of Morbidity

To meet this responsibility, the Interim Commission appointed the Expert Committee for the Preparation of the Sixth Decennial Revision of the International Lists of Diseases and Causes of Death.

This Committee, taking full account of prevailing opinion concerning morbidity and mortality classification, reviewed and revised the above-mentioned proposed classification which had been prepared by the United States Committee on Joint Causes of Death.

The resulting classification was circulated to national governments preparing morbidity and mortality statistics for comments and suggestions under the title, *International Classification of Diseases, Injuries, and Causes of Death.* The Expert Committee considered the replies and prepared a revised version incorporating such changes as appeared to improve the utility and acceptability of the classification. The Committee also compiled a list of diagnostic terms to appear under each title of the classification. Furthermore, a subcommittee was appointed to prepare a comprehensive alphabetical index of diagnostic statements classified to the appropriate category of the classification.

The Committee also considered the structure and uses of special lists of causes for tabulation and publication of morbidity and mortality statistics and studied other problems related to the international comparability of mortality statistics, such as form of medical certificate and rules for classification.

The International Conference for the Sixth Revision of the International Lists of Diseases and Causes of Death was convened in Paris from 26 to 30 April 1948 by the Government of France under the terms of the agreement signed at the close of the Fifth Revision Conference in 1938. Its secretariat was entrusted jointly to the competent French authorities and to the World Health Organization, which had carried out the preparatory work under the terms of the arrangement concluded by the governments represented at the International Health Conference in 1946 (*19*).

The Conference adopted the classification prepared by the Expert Committee as the Sixth Revision of the International Lists (*20*). It also considered other proposals of the Expert Committee concerning the compilation, tabulation and publication of morbidity and mortality statistics. The Conference approved the International Form of Medical Certificate of Cause of Death, accepted the underlying cause of death as the main cause to be tabulated, and endorsed the rules for selecting the underlying cause of death as well as the special lists for tabulation of morbidity and mortality data. It further recommended that the World Health Assembly should adopt regulations under *Article 21(b)* of the WHO Constitution to guide Member States in compiling morbidity and mortality statistics in accordance with the International Statistical Classification.

In 1948, the First World Health Assembly endorsed the report of the Sixth Revision Conference and adopted World Health Organization Regulations No. 1, prepared on the basis of the recommendations of the Conference. The International Classification, including the Tabular List of Inclusions defining the content of the categories, was incorporated, together with the form of the medical certificate of cause of death, the rules for classification and the special lists for tabulation, into the *Manual of the International Statistical Classification of Diseases, Injuries, and Causes of Death* (*21*). The Manual consisted of two volumes, Volume 2 being an alphabetical index of diagnostic terms coded to the appropriate categories.The Sixth Decennial Revision Conference marked the beginning of a new era in international vital and health statistics. Apart from approving a comprehensive list for both mortality and morbidity and agreeing on international rules for selecting the underlying cause of death, it recommended the adoption of a comprehensive programme of international cooperation in the field of vital and health statistics. An important item in this programme was the recommendation that governments establish national committees on vital and health statistics to coordinate the statistical activities in the country, and to serve as a link between the national statistical institutions and the World Health Organization. It was further envisaged that such national committees would, either singly or in cooperation with other national committees, study statistical problems of public health importance and make the results of their investigations available to WHO.

6.7   The Seventh and Eighth Revisions

The International Conference for the Seventh Revision of the International Classification of Diseases was held in Paris under the auspices of WHO in February 1955 (22). In accordance with a recommendation of the WHO Expert Committee on Health Statistics, this revision was limited to essential changes and amendments of errors and inconsistencies (23).

The Eighth Revision Conference convened by WHO met in Geneva, from 6 to 12 July 1965 (24). This revision was more radical than the Seventh but left unchanged the basic structure of the Classification and the general philosophy of classifying diseases, whenever possible, according to their etiology rather than a particular manifestation.

During the years that the Seventh and Eighth Revisions of the ICD were in force, the use of the ICD for indexing hospital medical records increased rapidly and some countries prepared national adaptations which provided the additional detail needed for this application of the ICD.

6.8   The Ninth Revision

The International Conference for the Ninth Revision of the International Classification of Diseases, convened by WHO, met in Geneva from 30 September to 6 October 1975 (25). In the discussions leading up to the conference, it had originally been intended that there should be little change other than updating of the classification. This was mainly because of the expense of adapting data-processing systems each time the classification was revised. There had been an enormous growth of interest in the ICD and ways had to be found of responding to this, partly by modifying the classification itself and partly by introducing special coding provisions. A number of representations were made by specialist bodies which had become interested in using the ICD for their own statistics. Some subject areas in the classification were regarded as inappropriately arranged and there was considerable pressure for more detail and for adaptation of the classification to make it more relevant for the evaluation of medical care, by classifying conditions to the chapters concerned with the part of the body affected rather than to those dealing with the underlying generalized disease. At the other end of the scale, there were representations from countries and areas where a detailed and sophisticated classification was irrelevant, but which nevertheless needed a classification based on the ICD in order to assess their progress in health care and in the control of disease.

The final proposals presented to and accepted by the Conference retained the basic structure of the ICD, although with much additional detail at the level of the four-digit subcategories, and some optional five-digit subdivisions. For the benefit of users not requiring such detail, care was taken to ensure that the categories at the three-digit level were appropriate.

For the benefit of users wishing to produce statistics and indexes oriented towards medical care, the Ninth Revision included an optional alternative method of classifying diagnostic statements, including information about both an underlying general disease and a manifestation in a particular organ or site. This system became known as the dagger and asterisk system and is retained in the Tenth Revision. A number of other technical innovations were included in the Ninth Revision, aimed at increasing its flexibility for use in a variety of situations.

The Twenty-ninth World Health Assembly, noting the recommendations of the International Conference for the Ninth Revision of the International Classification of Diseases, approved the publication, for trial purposes, of supplementary classifications of Impairments and Handicaps and of Procedures in Medicine as supplements to, but not as integral parts of, the International Classification of Diseases. The Conference also made recommendations on a number of related technical subjects: coding rules for mortality were amended slightly and rules for the selection of a single cause for tabulation of morbidity were introduced for the first time; definitions and recommendations for statistics in the field of perinatal mortality were amended and extended and a certificate of causes of perinatal death was recommended; countries were encouraged to do further work on multiple-condition coding and analysis, but no formal methods were recommended; and a new basic tabulation list was produced.

6.9   Preparations for the Tenth Revision

Even before the Conference for the Ninth Revision, WHO had been preparing for the Tenth Revision. It had been realized that the great expansion in the use of the ICD necessitated a thorough rethinking of its structure and an effort to devise a stable and flexible classification, which should not require fundamental revision for many years to come. The WHO Collaborating Centres for Classification of Diseases (see Volume 1) were consequently called upon to experiment with models of alternative structures for ICD-10.

It had also become clear that the established ten-year interval between revisions was too short. Work on the revision process had to start before the current version of the ICD had been in use long enough to be thoroughly evaluated, mainly because the necessity to consult so many countries and organizations made the process a very lengthy one. The Director-General of WHO therefore wrote to the Member States and obtained their agreement to postpone until 1989 the Tenth Revision Conference, which was originally scheduled for 1985 and to delay the introduction of the Tenth Revision which would have been due in 1989. In addition to permitting experimentation with alternative models for the structure of the ICD, this allowed time for the evaluation of ICD-9, for example through meetings organized by some of the WHO Regional Offices and through a survey organized at headquarters.

An extensive programme of work followed which culminated in the Tenth Revision of the ICD and is described in the Report of the International Conference for the Tenth Revision of the International Classification of Diseases, reproduced in Volume 1.

7. Appendices

7.1   List of conditions unlikely to cause death

Code	Category or subcategory
A31.1	Cutaneous mycobacterial infection
A42.8	Other forms of cutaneous actinomycosis
A60.0	Herpesviral infection of genitalia and urogenital tract
A71.0–A71.9	Trachoma
A74.0	Chlamydial conjunctivitis
B00.2	Herpesviral gingivostomatitis
B00.5	Herpesviral ocular disease
B00.8	Herpesviral whitlow
B07	Viral warts
B08.1	Molluscum contagiosum
B08.8	Foot and mouth disease
B30.0–B30.9	Viral conjunctivitis
B35.0–B35.9	Dermatophytosis
B36.0–B36.9	Other superficial mycoses
B85.0–B85.4	Pediculosis and phthiriasis
F45.3–F45.9	Somatoform disorders
F50.1, F50.3–F50.9	Eating disorders
F51.0–F51.9	Nonorganic sleep disorders
F52.0–F52.9	Sexual dysfunction, not caused by organic disorder or disease
F60.0–F60.9	Specific personality disorders
F61	Mixed and other personality disorders
F62.0–F62.9	Enduring personality changes, not attributable to brain damage and disease
F63.0–F63.9	Habit and impulse disorders
F64.0–F64.9	Gender identity disorders
F65.0–F65.9	Disorders of sexual preference
F66.0–F66.9	Psychological and behavioural disorders associated with sexual development and orientation
F68.0–F68.9	Other disorders of adult personality and behaviour
F69	Unspecified disorder of adult personality and behaviour

Code	Category or subcategory
F95.0–F95.9	Tic disorders
F98.0–F98.9	Other behavioural and emotional disorders with an onset usually occurring in childhood and adolescence
G43.0–G43.2, G43.8–G43.9	Migraine, except complicated migraine (G43.3)
G44.0–G44.2	Other headache syndromes
G45.0–G45.9	Transient cerebral ischaemic attacks and related syndromes
G50.0–G50.9	Disorders of trigeminal nerve
G51.0–G51.9	Facial nerve disorders
G54.0–G54.9	Nerve root and plexus disorders
G56.0–G56.9	Mononeuropathies of upper limb
G57.0–G57.9	Mononeuropathies of lower limb
G58.7	Mononeuritis multiplex
H00.0–H00.1	Hordeolum and chalazion
H01.0–H01.9	Other inflammation of eyelid
H02.0–H02.9	Other disorders of eyelid
H04.0–H04.9	Disorders of lacrimal system
H10.0–H10.9	Conjunctivitis
H11.0–H11.9	Other disorders of conjunctiva
H15.0–H15.9	Disorders of sclera
H16.0–H16.9	Keratitis
H17.0–H17.9	Corneal scars and opacities
H18.0–H18.9	Other disorders of cornea
H20.0–H20.9	Iridocyclitis
H21.0–H21.9	Other disorders of iris and ciliary body
H25.0–H25.9	Senile cataract
H26.0–H26.9	Other cataract
H27.0–H27.9	Other disorders of lens
H30.0–H30.9	Chorioretinal inflammation
H31.0–H31.9	Other disorders of choroid
H33.0–H33.5	Retinal detachments and breaks
H34.0–H34.9	Retinal vascular occlusions
H35.0–H35.9	Other retinal disorders
H40.0–H40.9	Glaucoma
H43.0–H43.9	Disorders of vitreous body
H46	Optic neuritis
H47.0–H47.7	Other disorders of optic (2nd) nerve and visual pathways
H49.0–H49.9	Paralytic strabismus
H50.0–H50.9	Other strabismus

Code	Category or subcategory
H51.0–H51.9	Other disorders of binocular movement
H52.0–H52.7	Disorders of refraction and accommodation
H53.0–H53.9	Visual disturbances
H54.0–H54.9	Blindness and low vision
H55	Nystagmus and other irregular eye movements
H57.0–H57.9	Other disorders of eye and adnexa
H59.0–H59.9	Postprocedural disorders of eye and adnexa, not elsewhere classified
H60.0–H60.9	Otitis externa
H61.0–H61.9	Other disorders of external ear
H80.0–H80.9	Otosclerosis
H83.3–H83.9	Other diseases of inner ear
H90.0–H90.8	Conductive and sensorineural hearing loss
H91.0–H91.9	Other hearing loss
H92.0–H92.2	Otalgia and effusion of ear
H93.0–H93.9	Other disorders of ear, not elsewhere classified
J00	Acute nasopharyngitis [common cold]
J06.0–J06.9	Acute upper respiratory infections of multiple and unspecified sites
J30.0–J30.4	Vasomotor and allergic rhinitis
J33.0–J33.9	Nasal polyp
J34.2	Deviated nasal septum
J35.0–J35.9	Chronic disease of tonsils and adenoids
K00.0–K00.9	Disorders of tooth development and eruption
K01.0–K01.1	Embedded and impacted teeth
K02.0–K02.9	Dental caries
K03.0–K03.9	Other diseases of hard tissues of teeth
K04.0–K04.9	Diseases of pulp and periapical tissues
K05.0–K05.6	Gingivitis and periodontal diseases
K06.0–K06.9	Other disorders of gingiva and edentulous alveolar ridge
K07.0–K07.9	Dentofacial anomalies (including malocclusion)
K08.0–K08.9	Other disorders of teeth and supporting structures
K09.0–K09.9	Cyst of oral region, not elsewhere classified
K10.0–K10.9	Other diseases of jaws
K11.0–K11.9	Diseases of salivary glands
K14.0–K14.9	Diseases of tongue
L01.0–L01.1	Impetigo (for infants over 1 year of age)

Code	Category or subcategory
L03.0	Cellulitis of finger and toe
L04.0–L04.9	Acute lymphadenitis
L05.0–L05.9	Pilonidal cyst
L08.0–L08.8	Other local infections of skin and subcutaneous tissue
L20.0–L20.9	Atopic dermatitis
L21.0–L21.9	Seborrhoeic dermatitis
L22	Diaper [napkin] dermatitis
L23.0–L23.9	Allergic contact dermatitis
L24.0–L24.9	Irritant contact dermatitis
L25.0–L25.9	Unspecified contact dermatitis
L28.0–L28.2	Lichen simplex chronicus and prurigo
L29.0–L29.9	Pruritus
L30.0–L30.9	Other dermatitis
L41.0–L41.9	Parapsoriasis
L42	Pityriasis rosea
L43.0–L43.9	Lichen planus
L44.0–L44.9	Other papulosquamous disorders
L55.0–L55.1, L55.8–L55.9	Sunburn, except sunburn of third degree (L55.2)
L56.0–L56.9	Other acute skin changes due to ultraviolet radiation
L57.0–L57.9	Skin changes due to chronic exposure to nonionizing radiation
L58.0–L58.9	Radiodermatitis
L59.0–L59.9	Other disorders of skin and subcutaneous tissue related to radiation
L60.0–L60.9	Nail disorders
L63.0–L63.9	Alopecia areata
L64.0–L64.9	Androgenic alopecia
L65.0–L65.9	Other nonscarring hair loss
L66.0–L66.9	Cicatricial alopecia [scarring hair loss]
L67.0–L67.9	Hair colour and hair shaft abnormalities
L68.0–L68.9	Hypertrichosis
L70.0–L70.9	Acne
L72.0–L72.9	Follicular cysts of skin and subcutaneous tissue
L73.0–L73.9	Other follicular disorders
L74.0–L74.9	Eccrine sweat disorders
L75.0–L75.9	Aprocrine sweat disorders
L80	Vitiligo
L81.0–L81.9	Other disorders of pigmentation

Code	Category or subcategory
L83	Acanthosis nigricans
L84	Corns and callosities
L85.0–L85.9	Other epidermal thickening
L87.0–L87.9	Transepidermal elimination disorders
L90.0–L90.9	Atrophic disorders of skin
L91.0–L91.9	Hypertrophic disorders of skin
L92.0–L92.9	Granulomatous disorders of skin and subcutaneous tissue
L94.0–L94.9	Other localized connective tissue disorders
L98.0–L98.3, L98.5-L95.9	Other disorders of skin and subcutaneous tissue, not elsewhere classified
M20.0–M20.6	Acquired deformities of fingers and toes
M21.0–M21.9	Other acquired deformities of limbs
M22.0–M22.9	Disorders of patella
M23.0–M23.9	Internal derangement of knee
M24.0–M24.9	Other specific joint derangements
M25.0–M25.9	Other joint disorders, not elsewhere classified
M35.3	Polymyalgia rheumatica
M40.0–M40.5	Kyphosis and lordosis
M43.6	Torticollis, unspecified
M43.8–M43.9	Other and unspecified deforming dorsopathies
M48.0	Spinal stenosis (except for the cervical region)
M53.0–M53.9	Other dorsopathies, not elsewhere classified
M54.0–M54.9	Dorsalgia
M60.0–M60.9	Myositis
M65.0–M65.9	Synovitis and tenosynovitis
M66.0–M66.5	Spontaneous rupture of synovium and tendon
M67.0–M67.9	Other disorders of synovium and tendon
M70.0–M70.9	Soft tissue disorders related to use, overuse and pressure
M71.0–M71.9	Other bursopathies
M72.5	Fasciitis, not elsewhere classified
M75.0–M75.9	Shoulder lesions
M76.0–M76.9	Enthesopathies of lower limb, excluding foot
M77.0–M77.9	Other enthesopathies
M79.0–M79.9	Other soft tissue disorders, not elsewhere classified
M95.0–M95.9	Other acquired deformities of musculoskeletal system and connective tissue
M99.0–M99.9	Biomechanical lesions, not elsewhere classified

Code	Category or subcategory
N39.3	Stress incontinence
N46	Male infertility
N47	Redundant prepuce, phimosis, and paraphimosis
N60.0–N60.9	Benign mammary dysplasia
N84.0–N84.9	Polyp of female genital tract
N85.0–N85.9	Other noninflammatory disorders of uterus, except cervix
N86	Erosion and ectropion of cervix uteri
N87.0–N87.9	Dysplasia of cervix uteri
N88.0–N88.9	Other noninflammatory disorders of cervix uteri
N89.0–N89.9	Other noninflammatory disorders of vagina
N90.0–N90.9	Other noninflammatory disorders of vulva and perineum
N91.0–N91.5	Absent, scanty, and rare menstruation
N92.0–N92.9	Excessive, frequent, and irregular menstruation
N93.0–N93.9	Other abnormal uterine and vaginal bleeding
N94.0–N94.9	Pain and other conditions associated with female genital organs and menstrual cycle
N96	Habitual aborter
N97.0–N97.9	Female infertility
Q10.0–Q10.7	Congenital malformations of eyelid, lacrimal apparatus and orbit
Q11.0–Q11.3	Anophthalmos, microphthalmos and macrophthalmos
Q12.0–Q12.9	Congenital lens malformations
Q13.0–Q13.9	Congenital malformations of anterior segment of eye
Q14.0–Q14.9	Congenital malformations of posterior segment of eye
Q15.0–Q15.9	Other congenital malformations of eye
Q16.0–Q16.9	Congenital malformations of ear causing impairment of hearing
Q17.0–Q17.9	Other congenital malformations of ear
Q18.0–Q18.9	Other congenital malformations of face and neck
Q38.1	Tongue tie
Q65.0–Q65.9	Congenital deformities of hip
Q66.0–Q66.9	Congenital deformities of feet

Code	Category or subcategory
Q67.0–Q67.8	Congenital musculoskeletal deformities of head, face, spine and chest
Q68.0–Q68.8	Other congenital musculoskeletal deformities
Q69.0–Q69.9	Polydactyly
Q70.0–Q70.9	Syndactyly
Q71.0–Q71.9	Reduction defects of upper limb
Q72.0–Q72.9	Reduction defects of lower limb
Q73.0–Q73.8	Reduction defects of unspecified limb
Q74.0–Q74.9	Other congenital malformations of limb(s)
Q80.0–Q80.3, Q80.8–Q80.9	Congenital ichthyosis, except Harlequin fetus (Q80.4)
Q81.0	Epidermolysis bullosa simplex
Q81.2–Q81.9	Other forms of epidermolysis bullosa, except epidermolysis bullosa letalis (Q81.1)
Q82.0–Q82.9	Other congenital malformations of skin
Q83.0–Q83.9	Congenital malformations of breast
Q84.0–Q84.9	Other congenital malformations of integument
S00.0–S00.9	Superficial injury of head
S05.0, S05.1, S05.8	Superficial injuries (any type) of eye and orbit (any part)
S10.0–S10.9	Superficial injury of neck
S20.0–S20.8	Superficial injury of thorax
S30.0–S30.9	Superficial injury of abdomen, lower back and pelvis
S40.0–S40.9	Superficial injury of shoulder and upper arm
S50.0–S50.9	Superficial injury of forearm
S60.0–S60.9	Superficial injury of wrist and hand
S70.0–S70.9	Superficial injury of hip and thigh
S80.0–S80.9	Superficial injury of lower leg
S90.0–S90.9	Superficial injury of ankle and foot
T09.0	Superficial injury of trunk, level unspecified
T11.0	Superficial injury of upper limb, level unspecified
T13.0	Superficial injury of lower limb, level unspecified
T14.0	Superficial injury of unspecified body region
T20.1	Burn of first degree of head and neck
T21.1	Burn of first degree of trunk
T22.1	Burn of first degree of shoulder and upper limb, except wrist and hand

Code	Category or subcategory
T23.1	Burn of first degree of wrist and hand
T24.1	Burn of first degree of hip and lower limb except ankle and foot
T25.1	Burn of first degree of ankle and foot

References

1. *International classification of diseases for oncology* (ICD-O), second ed. Geneva, World Health Organization, 1990.
2. *Systematized nomenclature of medicine* (SNOMED). Chicago, College of American Pathologists, 1976.
3. *Manual of tumor nomenclature and coding* (MOTNAC). New York, American Cancer Society, 1968.
4. *Systematized nomenclature of pathology* (SNOP). Chicago, College of American Pathologists, 1965.
5. *The ICD-10 classification of mental and behavioural disorders: clinical descriptions and diagnostic guidelines.* Geneva, World Health Organization, 1992.
6. *International classification of procedures in medicine* (ICPM). Vols 1 and 2. Geneva, World Health Organization, 1978.
7. *International classification of impairments, disabilities, and handicaps. A manual of classification relating to the consequences of disease.* Geneva, World Health Organization, 1980.
8. *International Nomenclature of Diseases.* Geneva, Council for International Organizations of Medical Sciences and World Health Organization; for details of individual volumes, see text.
9. *Sixteenth annual report.* London, Registrar General of England and Wales, 1856, App. p. 73.
10. Knibbs G.H. The International Classification of Disease and Causes of Death and its revision. *Medical journal of Australia*, 1929, 1:2-12.
11. Greenwood M. *Medical statistics from Graunt to Farr.* Cambridge, Cambridge University Press, 1948.
12. *First annual report.* London, Registrar General of England and Wales, 1839, p. 99.
13. Bertillon J. Classification of the causes of death (abstract). In: *Transactions of the 15th International Congress on Hygiene Demography*. Washington, 1912.
14. *Bulletin of the Institute of International Statistics*, 1900, 12:280.
15. Roesle E. *Essai d'une statistique comparative de la morbidité devant servir à établir les listes spéciales des causes de morbidité.* Geneva, League of Nations Health Organization, 1928 (document C.H. 730)
16. *International list of causes of death.* The Hague, International Statistical Institute, 1940.
17. Medical Research Council, Committee on Hospital Morbidity Statistics. *A provisional classification of diseases and injuries for use in compiling morbidity statistics.* London, Her Majesty's Stationery Office, 1944 (Special Report Series No. 248).

18. US Public Health Service, Division of Public Health Methods. *Manual for coding causes of illness according to a diagnosis code for tabulating morbidity statistics.* Washington, Government Publishing Office, 1944 (Miscellaneous Publication No. 32).
19. *Official Records of the World Health Organization,* 1948, 11, 23.
20. *Official Records of the World Health Organization,* 1948, 2, 110.
21. *Manual of the international statistical classification of diseases, injuries, and causes of death. Sixth revision.* Geneva, World Health Organization, 1949.
22. *Report of the International Conference for the Seventh Revision of the International Lists of Diseases and Causes of Death.* Geneva, World Health Organization, 1955 (unpublished document WHO/HA/7 Rev. Conf./17 Rev. 1.
23. *Third Report of the Expert Committee on Health Statistics.* Geneva, World Health Organization, 1952 (WHO Technical Report Series, No. 53).
24. *Report of the International Conference for the Eighth Revision of the International Classification of Diseases.* Geneva, World Health Organization, 1965 (unpublished document WHO/ICD9/74.4.
25. *Manual of the international statistical classification of diseases, injuries, and causes of death,* Volume 1. Geneva, World Health Organization, 1977.

Index